I dedicate this book to the original Tuxedo Warrior and master of Fitness on the Move™: Cliff Twemlow.

Fitness on the Move
Exercise Effectively Anywhere, Anytime.

Published by

MajorVision International

2017

Approved by The World Isometric Exercise Association

www.TWiEA.com

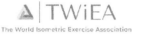

The World Isometric Exercise Association

Copyright and Trademark Notice
© 2017 Brian Sterling-Vete and Helen Renée Wuorio
All Rights Reserved

All material in this book is the property of, copyrighted, and trademarked to Brian Sterling-Vete and Helen Renée Wuorio, and/or MajorVision Ltd, unless otherwise stated, AE&OE. Copyright and other intellectual property laws protect these materials. Reproduction, distribution, or transmission of the materials, in whole or in part, in any manner, without the prior written consent of the copyright holder is prohibited and is a violation of national and international copyright law.

The following names, exercises, and workout systems are the property of, copyright, and trademarked to Brian Sterling-Vete and Helen Renée, and/or MajorVision Ltd. ISOfitness™, The 70 Second Difference™, Adaptive Response™, The 1664 Workout™, The 1664 Workout Challenge™, Zero Footprint Workout™, ZFW™, Fitness on the Move™, FOM™, The ISO90™ Course, ISO90™, The SSASS Workout™, SSASS™, Dynamic Flexation™, The Bullworker Bible™, The Bullworker 90™, The Bullworker Compendium™, Workout at Work™, Doorway to Strength™, The TRISO90™ Course, TRISOmetrics™, The ISOmetric Bible™, Brian Sterling-Vete's Mental Martial Arts™, Tuxedo Warriors™, The Tuxedo Warrlor™, The Pike™, The Beast of Kane™, Being American Married to a Brit, and Paranormal Investigation - The Black Book of Scientific Ghost Hunting and How to Investigate Paranormal Phenomena™, The Haunting of Lilford Hall™.

Artwork and design: **WWW.MAJORVISION.COM**
WWW.MAJORVISION.COM – WWW.TWiEA.COM

Contents

Important General Safety and Health Guidelines

1. **The Beginning**
2. **Fitness on the Move™ and the Zero Footprint Exercise™ Concept**
3. **Exercise Science Overview**
   - The Basic Types of Resistance Exercise
   - Isometric Overview
   - Isometric Exercise Science
   - The Standard Isometric Contraction
   - Workout Intensity
   - Technically, How Does a Muscle Grow?
   - Rest Time Between Exercises
   - Dynamic Flexation™
   - Isometric Exercises and Blood Pressure
   - Rest and Recovery
   - Adequate Nutrition is Vital
   - Strength, Stamina, Endurance, and Resilience
   - Biceps, Supination, and Strong Arms
4. **All Things Iso-Bow®**
   - Securing The Iso-Bow® With Your Feet
   - Shortening The Iso-Bow®
5. **About the Exercise Model**
   - The Author and an Isometric Experiment
6. **Important Stuff Before You Begin**
7. **Fitness on the Move™ Exercises Resources**
8. **Conclusion**

www.MajorVsion.com

Important General Safety and Health Guidelines

This section entitled, "Important General Safety and Health Guidelines," pertains to The ISOfitness™ Exercise System, and all books and publications about it not limited to but including The ISO90™ Course, Fitness on the Move™, The 70 Second Difference™, The Bullworker Bible™, the Sixty Second Ass Workout™, The Bullworker 90™ Course, The Bullworker Compendium™, Workout at Work™, The Doorway to Strength™, The TRISO90™ Course, TRISOmetric™, TRISOmetrics™, ISOmetrics, The ISOmetric Bible™, the Iso-Bow® System, recommendations, suggestions, coaching, and advice, either written, verbal, in audio format, on video, written, or given, implied, or suggested the authors, from Brian Sterling-Vete, Helen Renée Wuorio, and the works thereof.

You should never begin any kind of sport, exercise system, workout plan, or diet modification, including everything contained in this book and any books mentioned in the beginning paragraph above unless you have consulted with and have the full approval of your medical doctor.

Your physician can accurately assess your current health status, and your ability to perform the exercises in the book and/or course. This is particularly important if you have any known or unknown pre-existing health issues, are pregnant, or believe that you may have other serious health conditions.

You must always have absolute approval from your physician before starting. Please show all the material in the above courses, books, video/audio, online material, and their content to your physician and get their approval before you start.

All exercises, suggestions, recommendations, instructions, exercise plans, and dietary recommendations, either given or implied, are intended only as a reference, and they are no substitute for a qualified professional personal coach who can help you plan an exercise and diet program appropriate for your age and physical condition. Never overexert yourself when performing any exercise.

Stop exercising immediately and consult your doctor if you ever experience any pain, irregular heartbeat, shortness of breath, tightness in your chest/arms/fingers, faintness, nausea, or feelings of dizziness. Then consult your doctor and/or call the EMS immediately.

The exercises, courses, plans, and dietary recommendations in this book together with all those mentioned in all the books, general publications, online material, and videos mentioned in the names in paragraph 1 of this section, are not intended for use by children. Keep all exercise equipment out of the reach of children.

Always inspect any exercise equipment, and/or any/all other improvised or specifically made exercise equipment/materials, doors, door jambs, door frames, and anything else you use before each use to ensure its proper operation and to ensure that it is undamaged and safe. Do not use it unless all parts are free from wear, and it is functioning properly. Care should always be taken to avoid serious injury using any/all exercise equipment and in all items, people, books, and courses mentioned in paragraph 1 of this section.

Care should always be taken when getting into all exercise positions, on and off the floor, on and off chairs, on and off benches, on and off any other surface that might be used for exercise, including pieces of furniture, and in the use of all exercised equipment, either purpose-made or improvised.

The creators, writers, instructors, originators, and owners of The Bullworker 90™ Course, The ISO 90 Course™, The TRISO 90™ Course, and all other courses, publications on video, audio, and in print, together with the courses, and websites, owned, originated, and created by the copyright holders and the ISOfitness™ team, including all books, courses, and people mentioned in paragraph 1 of this section, accept no responsibility whatsoever for any injury, harm, damage, illness, harm, damage to property, or any other negative health-related condition which may occur as a direct, or indirect result of following these courses, recommendations, suggestions, diagrams, pictures, videos, or while performing any exercises in these or any related other related material/publication/s.

For additional general information, we also recommend that you check reputable accredited medical advice sites, such as the two listed below.

The National Health Service in the United Kingdom, online at:
https://www.nhs.uk/Livewell/fitness/pages/physical-activity-guidelines-for-adults.aspx

In the USA, The Mayo Clinic online:
http://www.mayoclinic.org/healthy-lifestyle/fitness/in-depth/exercise/art-20047414

Chapter 1: The Beginning...

"Fitness on the Move™" is a concept I had as far back as the late 1970s. After I had been exercising for several years, as well as teaching martial arts, I decided to attend university to begin studying exercise science formally. However, with the added pressure of studying at university added to my already busy sports and social life, there were times when it appeared there just were not enough hours in a day to include an effective regular exercise routine. To make ends meet financially in those days I was eventually forced to add an extra job to an already tightly packed schedule. The extra job was that of a Tuxedo Warrior, or nightclub bouncer as it is more commonly known. Therefore, the additional strain of working late into the night sometimes made it impossible to exercise effectively on both the day I worked and the day afterwards. One of the problems, apart from always needing more sleep, was that during the times when I was free to exercise, the gym was not open, and I did not own much exercise equipment other than an original Bullworker®. The Bullworker® was a great piece of equipment, and as with all new "toys," when I first got one, I used it regularly and made some excellent gains as a result. Unfortunately, I never really took it too seriously, and foolishly used it only as an addition to my gym workouts, instead of following the instructions to the letter. As with all young people, when the next "bright and shiny" thing came along to distract me, I gave that my fullest attention and left the Bullworker® gathering dust in a corner. That was until I got to know a fellow Tuxedo Warrior a little better, a man by the name of Cliff Twemlow.

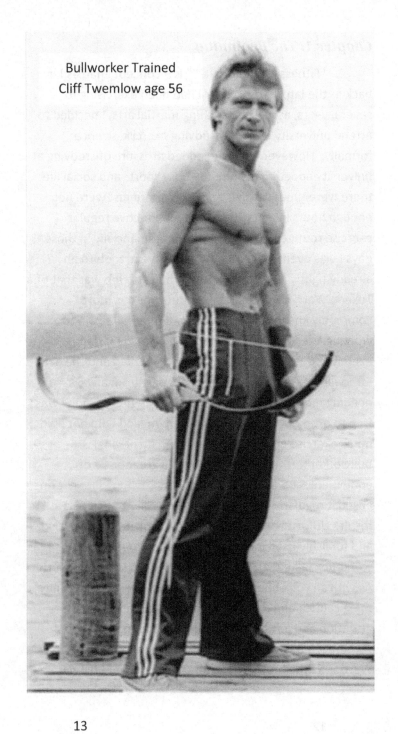
Bullworker Trained Cliff Twemlow age 56

Cliff was the head Tuxedo Warrior at Peter Stringfellow's Millionaire Nightclub in Manchester, and it was thanks to the manager of Manchester's Apollo Gym, John Cupello who'd introduced me to Cliff, who then helped me to get my badly needed extra job as a Tuxedo Warrior.

Cliff was a huge guy, with a deep chest, excellent definition, broad shoulders, and the classic 'V' shape of a typical heavy bodybuilder. A couple of years passed, and no matter what hours Cliff worked, he always seemed to stay in peak physical condition.

There were times when I thought that Cliff must secretly be some kind of super-human. This was because he was always fit, strong and immensely powerful, which were all essential elements if the job as a Tuxedo Warrior ever became physical – which it often did.

It was a quite different story for me though. I always seemed to be in some sort of time crunch crisis. I was struggling hard to make all my university, social, and work commitments fit together. Therefore, my gym sessions began to suffer. On occasions, I would even skip them altogether because I was just too tired, and I had no spare time anyway.

Suddenly, Cliff hit the proverbial jackpot. Unbeknownst to me, in his miraculously found spare time, Cliff had been working on his autobiography. He had called it "The Tuxedo Warrior," and not only had he managed to get it published, but he had also sold the movie rights to make a feature film from it!

In almost no time at all 'The Tuxedo Warrior' was being made into a Hollywood 'B' movie, with part of it filmed on location in Zimbabwe, Africa, as well as various other locations around the UK.

I was honoured to be given a few small roles in the movie as a 'martial arts stuntman' performing various fight scenes. These were my first small steps into the TV, film, and media industries. More importantly, this was the time when I discovered Cliff's secret of how he managed to stay in such great shape and maintain his incredible strength even without a gym. He had developed 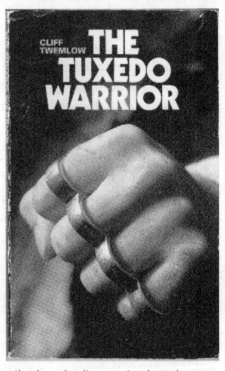 what could only be described as the 'improvised workout session' into an art form, thanks to isometric exercise.

This was when I found out that Cliff was a true devotee of the Bullworker® and isometric exercise in general. The difference between my experience with the Bullworker®, and how Cliff approached it was actually remarkably simple.

I originally tended to use the Bullworker®, and the isometric exercise system, purely as a means of getting a little extra exercise, and I did not take it seriously enough. Conversely, Cliff used the Bullworker® with the same level of dedication and intensity that someone would employ during a workout in a professional gym.

Cliff did not really understand the science of why isometric exercises worked so well, and even the university course of exercise science I was committed to at the time did not cover the subject of isometrics in much depth. It was not until I studied exercise science at much higher academic levels in later years that I would be able to study the real science of all things isometric.

At the time, all that we cared about was the fact that we both knew that the Bullworker® and isometric exercises worked exceptionally well. This was the "secret" of how Cliff had always managed to stay strong, muscular, and in great shape, even if there was no time to exercise in traditional ways in a gym.

One of the things which surprised me the most was how brief the isometric exercise sessions were, especially when compared to the long hours I used to spend exercising at the Apollo Gym.

I was also incredibly surprised to experience how powerful a properly executed isometric exercise could be. I found that when I used proper breathing control to ensure that I never held my breath during an exercise, and when I applied a high level of focused force and intensity, the results I got were easily equal to a long traditional gym session.

This was the point when I began to take a serious interest in isometric exercise, I also learned that the results I achieved from an isometric exercise session were directly proportional to the level of effort, force, and overall intensity I applied to that session.

I do not know why I found this so surprising at the time, I knew the same rule applied to my traditional gym workout sessions, but I had never made the connection to apply it to an isometric session. Perhaps it was my fault for always treating isometrics as some sort of novelty before the Eureka moment I had about them, thanks to Cliff Twemlow.

Isometric exercises were the answer I had been looking for. I then began using my Bullworker® with the same levels of intensity and commitment that Cliff employed during his workout sessions. Very soon, I found that I was getting remarkably similar results to Cliff. The brief, focused, and intense workout sessions using the Bullworker® and isometric exercises soon had me packing on even more muscle than I had gained from my traditional gym workouts in the past.

The isometric system worked EXCEPTIONALLY well. Furthermore, because the workout sessions were isometric, even a full-body workout only took minutes to perform! I suddenly found that I had acquired a 'time' dividend. Thanks to isometric exercise sessions I had all the time I needed to meet my university, social, and work commitments, and still stay strong, muscular, and fit!

In the years that followed, no matter what I did, and no matter where I travelled, my Bullworker® would always be with me. Isometrics would always be a particularly important part of my life from that time onwards.

Between the late 1970s and early 1990s, I made 11 movies with Cliff. Some of these were filmed in wild, remote, and exotic locations such as Africa, the Caribbean, Iceland, and the Mediterranean. I also found out just how long the days can be working in the movie industry, and

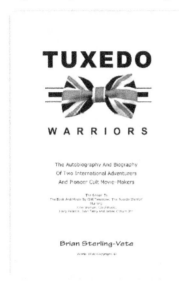

how an isometric workout is perhaps the only way possible to maintain an effective exercise routine under such circumstances. Since you are reading this book you have almost certainly read the summary about it before you bought it. In that summary, you will have read that a "Fitness on the Move™" workout was had on the deck of a ship in a storm. Cliff and I were sailing on a tramp steamer out of Barcelona and encountered a storm as we did so. I will not go into more detail here since the full story is told in the "Tuxedo Warriors" book which you will read more about in the "Other books by the same author" section at the end of this book.

From the time I first discovered the real power of a properly performed isometric workout, no matter how remote or isolated the location was, and no matter how long the movie-making day would be, the Bullworker® always travelled with us. More importantly. Isometric exercise would ensure that both Cliff and I would stay in peak physical condition.

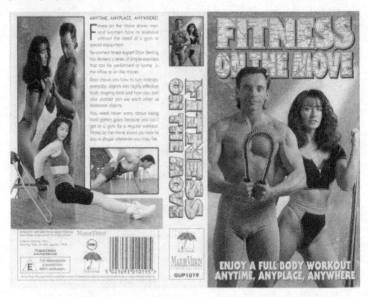

In 1990 I even produced an hour-long commercial exercise video entitled "Fitness on the Move™" and Cliff appeared in that, together with me and several other cast members. This was designed to show how easy it is to maintain an effective workout routine while travelling away from home for business or pleasure.

However, we deliberately did not include the Bullworker® or isometric exercises in it. This was for the simple reason that it would have been a particularly short video if we had! Instead, we chose to show how you can effectively use everyday objects as effective free-weight exercise tools. We also demonstrated how you can even use your luggage as effective dumbbells in a hotel room.

Interestingly, one of the cast members was also an excellent cameraman. When he was not in front of the camera doing exercises, he would swap with me and then operate the camera himself. Stuart Howell was a good friend, who also lodged at my house for several years.

Stuart went on from the "Fitness on the Move" video to operate the camera, a Steadicam, or as cinematographer on some major movies including: "The Legend of Tarzan," "London Has Fallen," Kingsman: "The Secret Service," "The Bourne Ultimatum," "Clash of the Titans," "Underworld," and "Fast & Furious 6," to name but a fraction of his prestigious list of credits.

Throughout my life, "Fitness on the Move™" would be part of my daily routine. Yes, I would occasionally spend time in various gyms, and I even used to own several commercial gyms myself. Exercising in a gym can be extremely productive, and there is also the fun social aspect to it all too.

However, it was all about freedom for me. The freedom of not having to always be near a gym because it was the only way I could get an effective regular workout. As a teenager, I had always dreamed about being freed from the time and commitment of working out in a gym, while still being able to grow serious muscle. My dream had eventually come true.

The only "problem" with the Bullworker®, if you can call it a "problem," is its physical size. Even though it is relatively compact by traditional gym equipment standards, it was still 36 inches in length and would not easily fit into a full-size suitcase, and you could just forget about trying to make it fit into carry-on-size luggage!

Naturally, it is possible to perform isometric exercises without a device such as a Bullworker®, but in my opinion, they are not as effective. There are several reasons why I feel this way, and my primary reasons are that it is just easier, more comfortable, and more biomechanically efficient with a device such as a Bullworker®.

The next stage of evolution in the "Fitness on the Move™" story would come many years later. It was when I was living temporarily in Minneapolis, Minnesota, in the United States, and one day a package arrived in the mail. It was from a good friend who had by that time bought the Bullworker® brand, and he had reinvented the device entirely.

John Hughes had given the Bullworker® the serious 21st-century make-over it had so desperately needed, and he had produced a much better device in every way. John had also produced a half-size version named: The Steel Bow®, complete with interchangeable springs offering different resistance levels, and a carry bag.

I bought one of the very first models John produced, and I took it with me on my business travels around the United States. It was much easier to travel with than a full-size Bullworker®, and it was possible to do almost as many exercises with it.

I opened the package John had sent to me in the mail and pulled out what at first appearance was nothing more than a small piece of webbing with handles, accompanied by a note. It simply read: "See what you think of this..."

I looked at what John had sent, and on closer examination, I now saw that it was a small figure-8 piece of webbing with the word Iso-Bow® embroidered on one side, and with a high-density foam handle at each end.

I also noted that it was very well made. In fact, the device was made to remarkably similar specifications as the webbing I used in climbing and abseiling. It was professional-grade, and so were the built-in handles.

In honesty, I played with the device for about half an hour, then I put it down on a dresser and did not even pick it up again until several months later. I simply texted John a reply saying, "Thank you, I will let you know..." and that was all.

Then one bright sunny day when I was exercising at home using John's newly redesigned Bullworker®, I was suddenly hit by the full realisation of what John had sent to me. He had sent me what I now consider to be "The Holy Grail" of exercise devices.

One that is small, light, and easily portable because a pair will fit into your pocket, it requires no maintenance or adjustment, and it can be used right out of the packet by anyone.

More importantly, without any adjustment, it can deliver a perfect level of workout for both a complete beginner and an advanced professional strength athlete! The Iso-Bow® was the device I had been waiting for to help make my wider concept of "Fitness on the Move™" become a reality.

Today, thanks to the genius of John Hughes in inventing the Iso-Bow®, together with the comprehensive print and video resources in the ISOfitness™ library, "Fitness on the Move" has not just finally 'come of age,' it has truly matured.

With just 2 Iso-Bow® devices® and an ISOfitness™ instruction coursebook, you can benefit from a high-level, gym-standard workout, anytime, anyplace, everywhere...

A footnote to the inspiration, Innovation, and Fitness on the Move motivation provided by the late pioneer filmmaker, Cliff Twemlow.

On the 27th of August 2023, a 120-minute award-winning documentary about the life and adventures of Cliff Twemlow was released with a red-carpet premiere on the IMAX screen at The Empire Cinema in Leicester Square in London.

My book, Tuxedo Warriors, was used as the primary template for the documentary that went on to premiere at major events in New York, Los Angeles, Austin Texas, Melbourn Australia, and Madrid, Spain.

The promo for the documentary can be found on YouTube at: https://youtu.be/6V-MWZDcccl

Chapter 2: Fitness on the Move™ and the Zero Footprint Exercise™ Concept

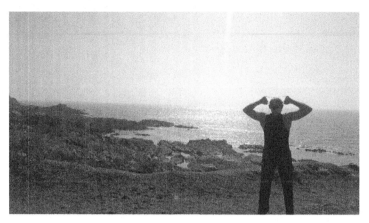

Fitness on the Move, Cornwall, England.

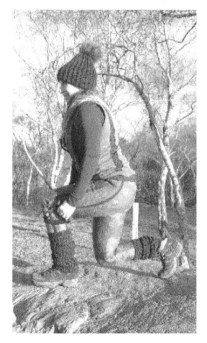

Lake District, England.

Now you know the background to the "Fitness on the Move™" concept, including how it started and how it has evolved. What does this all mean in practical terms? Surely most reasonably intelligent fitness enthusiasts are knowledgeable enough to piece together some sort of makeshift bodyweight-only resistance workout routine while they are travelling away from home and do not have access to a traditional gym. I am willing to bet that even at the time I was writing these words, and also at the time you are reading them, someone somewhere is having a workout in a hotel room or while travelling.

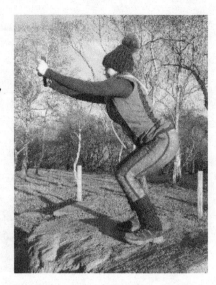

However, we believe that several important factors need to be considered to get the best workout possible in such circumstances. These are: 1) Is the workout routine the most time-efficient? 2) Is the type of exercise being performed able to deliver a high-intensity gym-standard workout? 3) Can the same exercises be performed in an almost Zero Footprint Exercise™ environment so they can be performed even as a passenger in

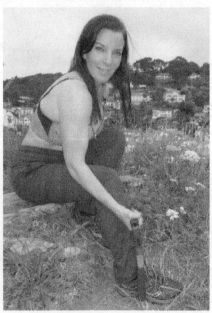

Cornwall, England.

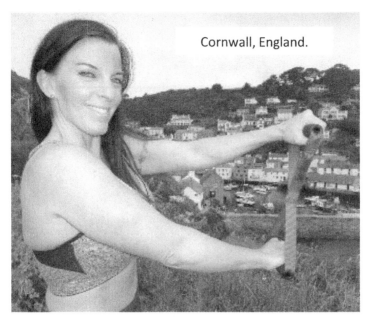

Cornwall, England.

a car or on a plane? 4) Are the exercise devices used lightweight, easily portable, and can be used by anybody at any level without adjustment? 5) Are you getting the maximum time and effort benefit from your choice of exercises and workout routine?

These are all excellent questions. In our experience, we also find that most people simply assume that the only viable

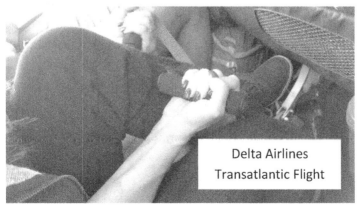

Delta Airlines Transatlantic Flight

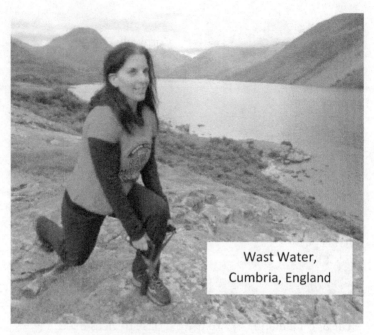

Wast Water, Cumbria, England

options for effective improvised workout routines revolve around the use of bodyweight-only callisthenic exercises.

They also assume that the only portable and effective exercise devices are things like elastic resistance bands and things of that nature. These things are good, and they can indeed deliver an excellent workout. More

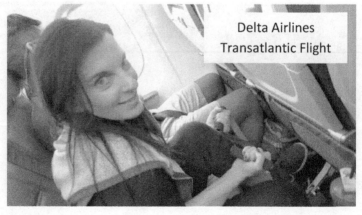

Delta Airlines Transatlantic Flight

importantly, it is always going to be far better to have any sort of workout rather than no workout at all.

Unfortunately, none of the above can deliver a true high-intensity, high-level, gym-standard workout in an extremely brief period, and an almost "Zero Footprint Workout™" environment. Our "Fitness on the Move™" combined with the Iso-Bow®, can do all those things exceptionally well.

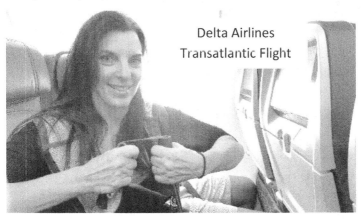

Delta Airlines Transatlantic Flight

All you need are three essential elements: 1) A pair of Iso-Bow® exercise devices 2) The knowledge contained in our books and course manuals 3) The motivation to exercise. If you have all three elements, then you can get strong, get fit, grow muscle, and build / tone/shape your body.

You may or may not already be aware that we have thoroughly tried and tested our "Fitness on the Move™" workout routines in all manner of confined, restricted, and unusual circumstances. We have benefitted from gym-standard, high-intensity exercise sessions while on transatlantic flights, on high-speed rail trips, as car

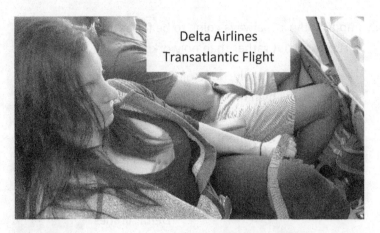

Delta Airlines Transatlantic Flight

passengers on road trips, on board a ship crossing the Mediterranean, on the ramparts of the famous Urquhart Castle on the banks of Loch Ness in Scotland, during a break from fell walking around Eskdale and Wast Water in the English Lake District, during several TV outside broadcasts while working with a famous US TV network, and while exploring the remote beaches and rocky coves in Cornwall, England which were used in the amazing "Poldark" TV series.

"Fitness on the Move™" exercises, together with the amazing Iso-Bow® device, have allowed us to maintain our workout routine wherever we have been travelling. It has also allowed us to benefit from a high-intensity pro-gym standard workout virtually anywhere.

We may have occasionally turned a few heads and attracted the attention of people who were nearby while we were exercising. However, almost all the attention was focused on how simple and effective our "Fitness on the Move™" exercises were.

We have even attracted the enthusiastic support of many airline pilots and cabin crew members who now use and love our ISOfitness™ system. One gentleman, a good friend who is a senior purser with a major airline, Rudy Finn, can only be described as a true 21st-century ISOfitness™ exercise evangelist! Well done, Rudy! We always look forward to seeing you regularly on our transatlantic flights.

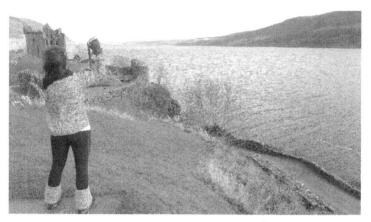

Loch Ness, Scotland.

We have chosen a comprehensive range of exercises that can be performed in an almost "Zero Footprint Workout™" environment while travelling. With these exercises, you will be able to exercise all the major muscle groups of the body.

For entirely practical purposes we decided that we would demonstrate how to perform some of the selected "Fitness on the Move™" exercises while seated as a passenger in an average family car. This is because it is probably a similar space to what you will have available to exercise in when travelling as a passenger in cars, trucks, ships, airliners, or trains. However, when we demonstrate exercises on beaches, on coastal paths, and by lakes, they can all be translated to be performed in a car, on a plane or in any other average vehicle. If you can stand up and or sit down, then, in theory, you can perform an isometric exercise session. This is a concept we call The Zero-Footprint™ Workout and it gives you the freedom to exercise anywhere, without traditional gym-based frontiers.

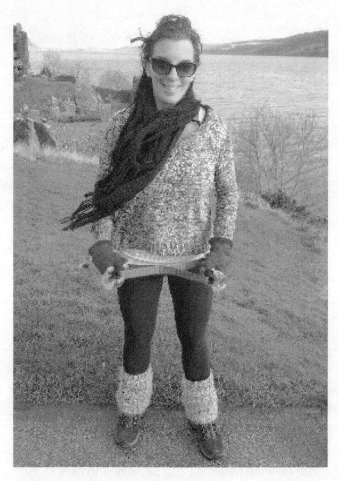

Loch Ness, Scotland.

Chapter 3: Exercise Science Overview

In this section, we will give a user-friendly overview of exercise science together with the features and benefits of various exercise techniques and concepts. For those who want more in-depth information about the science of isometric exercise and health and fitness in general, then we suggest that you also read our books The ISOmetric Bible™ and The 70 Second Difference™ books. Both are available on Amazon.

The Basic Types of Resistance Exercise

All muscle training falls into between two or three specific categories, depending upon how you break them down. In the most basic form, there are two types, either contraction with movement, or contraction without movement. Breaking them down a step further there become three categories, with one being isotonic, another isokinetic. Last but certainly not least, is isometric.

Isotonic training is all about movement with muscle shortening and lengthening during the lifting and lowering phases of the exercise. We know that the isotonic category can be broken down further into three parts. One part is the concentric contraction, which is the lifting phase of an exercise when the muscles shorten. Another is the eccentric phase which is the lowering part of an exercise when the muscles lengthen.

Lastly in this isotonic category is the isokinetic contraction. This is where the muscle changes in length during both the concentric and eccentric phases of the contraction, however, the velocity remains constant no matter how much force is applied during the exercises.

Then comes the isometric category. With an isometric exercise, there is no movement whatsoever. To help you envision this, I will take a random weight training or freehand callisthenic exercise such as a chest press because it can be performed either with movement OR without movement, as an isometric exercise.

For example, a barbell, a machine, or your bodyweight can be lifted and lowered to perform an exercise such as a barbell curl, this is called, isotonic exercise, callisthenics or simply exercise with movement.

To perform the same or similar exercise isometrically you would attempt to perform the same or similar biomechanically correct actions of a barbell curl, however, at a certain point, or points if multiple exercise points were being used, the curling movement would stop because an immovable object point had been reached.

At that point or points, you would apply an increasing level of force until you reach the desired target level as you attempt to perform the curling exercise against the immovable object.

At the desired isometric exercise point, a constant force is applied against the immovable object for 7 seconds which is the optimum isometric exercise time. The ideal basic isometric exercise point for general exercise is roughly at the mid-point when your muscles reach a stalemate working against each other or an immovable object. This is called a Standard isometric Contraction.

The harder you engage your muscles as you try to break the stalemate by lifting, pushing, or pulling, the stronger your muscles become. In doing so, you engage many more muscle fibres than normal as you attempt to move the immovable object and perform the curling exercise action.

Doors, desks, chairs, walls, and many other everyday items work well as immovable objects BUT the easiest and most used immovable object is typically yourself.

Isometric Overview

As you now know, isometric exercise does not involve any movement. Instead, the joint angle and the muscle length do not change during contraction. You also now know that 7 seconds is regarded as the optimum time to perform an isometric exercise.

However, almost everyone when exercising tends to count the exercise elapsed time much faster than real elapsed time. This means that it is easy not to reach the magic 7 seconds of the optimum isometric exercise time. Therefore, we always suggest aiming to perform the exercise for 10 seconds to ensure that the 7-second target is always reached even when under the stress of performing intense exercise.

Isometric exercise has been extensively scientifically researched and has been proven time and again to be a highly efficient way to build great strength and grow muscle. In fact, isometric exercise is probably one of the most thoroughly researched of all exercise systems.

However, it also remains one of the most misunderstood systems of exercise. This is almost certainly through fear, professional ignorance and purely financial reasons.

Several different techniques can be used in the isometric exercise system. Most of these techniques are highly advanced for use by competitive athletes, competitive martial arts practitioners, strength athletes and bodybuilders. Therefore, they have no application as part of a general isometric exercise session for the average person who simply wants to get generally stronger and fitter.

However, purely out of interest I will list them here in case any fitness enthusiasts, athletes or bodybuilders read this book and wish to try them. They are described in greater detail in our book called The Isometric Bible which is available on Amazon and in good bookstores. The most common and advanced isometric exercise techniques include the following:

- Standard Isometric Contraction
- Yielding Isometric Contraction
- Maximum Duration Isometrics
- Oscillatory Isometrics
- Impact Absorption Isometrics
- Explosive Isometrics, AKA: Ballistic Isometrics
- Static-Dynamic Isometric
- Isometric Contrast
- Functional Isometrics
- TRISOmetrics™

There are more than enough isometric exercises that can be performed without any equipment whatsoever to allow a total body workout routine to be completed relatively easily. These will typically be self-resisted isometric exercises, which are excellent. However, by using only minimal readily available equipment such as walking poles, golf clubs, martial arts belts, climbing ropes, scuba diving webbing weight belts, and broom handles etc. it is possible to greatly expand the number of exercises that can be performed.

It is also perfectly possible to adapt and use other readily available items such as tow ropes, steel chains, towels, and commonly found immobile objects such as sturdy fixed barrier railings, solid walls, solid doors, door frames, or parked vehicles to perform a complete isometric exercise routine. Again, these are all excellent improvised exercise tools that allow an expanded range of highly effective isometric exercises to be performed.

Using improvised exercise tools can yield an unexpected additional benefit. This is because it allows one to focus more and apply greater concentration to each exercise. This is particularly useful for those who are either completely new to, or who are relatively new to the isometric exercise system. We will explain more about what these can be later in the book.

One of the things we love about both the isometric and self-resisted systems of exercise is that as you get stronger through exercise, you can apply more force and intensity to your isometric or self-resisted exercises.

This, in turn, means that you can gradually increase the level of force you can safely apply to each exercise which will mean that the results and benefits you receive will grow in a compound way through regular daily use. This is what we call a natural Adaptive Response™ mechanism which is a useful aspect of our biology.

Isometric Exercise Science

Even until the mid-20th century, there was almost no scientific research that had been performed into the benefits of isometric exercise. We also know that before the first serious scientific research study, how people trained isometrically was typically by performing what we now call endurance isometrics.

Thankfully, isometric exercise has now been thoroughly scientifically researched and proven for several decades. I would estimate that there has probably been at least as much scientific research performed into isometric exercise as there has been into traditional resistance training.

The first major in-depth study into isometric exercise was performed at the world-famous Max Plank Institute in Dortmund, Germany. If you already have a reasonable knowledge of science, you will also know that the Max Plank Institute is a world-renowned centre of scientific excellence in many disciplines.

Between 1953 and 1958, one of the most extensive research studies was commissioned into isometric exercise science. These experiments are now considered by many to be the original gold standard of isometric exercise studies. The results were made widespread public knowledge in the resultant ground-breaking book, The Physiology of Strength, by Dr Theodor Hettinger - Research Fellow at the Max Plank

Institute. During that 5-year research period, Dr Hettinger and Dr Muller performed a widely reported, reputed 5,500 experiments, although this figure is almost certainly apocryphal because they would have had to perform a minimum of three experiments a day, every day for five years. Research suggests that the actual number of experiments performed by Hettinger and Muller was probably closer to 200, however, in wider studies at other institutions since that time, over 5,500 studies have almost certainly been completed. These were conducted on male and female volunteers from all walks of life and at every level of strength, fitness, and athletic ability. Perhaps what surprised people the most was how dramatic and impressive the results were gained from performing isometric exercises. Also, because the same or similar results were easily repeatable it made the data gained from the experiments exceptionally reliable.

The conclusion of the extensive studies proved beyond doubt the overall superiority of isometric exercise when it comes to building both strength and muscle, compared to traditional isotonic exercise methods. It also proved that the isometric system delivered these results much faster and with far less exercise than traditional resistance training. Another extremely interesting result emerged from the experiments. This was because it was not the length of time that an isometric exercise was held that produced the optimum results. Instead, it was the correct level of force applied for a very specific optimum time.

They found that performing only one daily isometric exercise for between 6 and 7 seconds, and at only two-thirds of an individual's maximum effort, could increase strength by an average of up to 5% per week. By any standards, strength gains of 5% in exchange for the expenditure of only 66%, or around two-thirds of an individual's maximum capacity, is an excellent result.

Perhaps even more amazingly, they discovered that after someone has performed a single 7-second training stimulus (exercise) per day, the muscle being exercised in that same position was no longer responsive to further gains. In other words, it did not matter how many more times you exercised the same muscle in the same position, there would be no further increase in muscle growth or strength. The only way to do this was to perform another isometric exercise at a different position only the ROM (Range Of Motion) of the limb being exercised. The scientific data about this can be referenced on pages 28 to 31 of Dr Theodor Hettinger's book, The Physiology of Strength.

In 2001, Nicolas Babault PhD of the University of Burgundy, Dijon, France, led a team of scientists to research and examine how many muscle fibres were activated, and how long they remained active during both traditional weight training and isometric training.

(*The scientific research paper is published: Nicolas Babault, Michel Pousson, Yves Ballay, and Jacques Van Hoecke - Groupe Analyse du Mouvement, Unite´ de Formation et de Recherche Sciences et Techniques des Activite´s Physiques et Sportives, Universite´ de Bourgogne, BP 27877, 21078 Dijon Cedex, France.*)

They discovered that when training intensely, and in near-perfect style, the levels of muscle activation during repetitions of optimum maximal weight training were between 89.7% during the concentric contraction, or when lifting a weight, and 88.3% during the eccentric contraction, or when lowering a weight. For practical purposes, an average of about 89% overall.

The study also revealed that during the lifting, or concentric part of the exercise, the maximum intramuscular tension only lasted for between 0.25 and 0.5 seconds. Which, for practical purposes is an average of about 1/3rd of a second during each isotonic repetition. This is because traditional isotonic resistance exercises naturally involve movement. They also have aspects of velocity and acceleration to consider in the overall equation. "Force" is only produced for a split second, to produce a maximal contraction of the muscle fibres.

The same research also showed that the level of muscle activation during isometric exercise was as high as 95.2% and that it lasted for the entire 7 to 10 seconds of each exercise. This is a huge increase over the 1/3rd of a second muscular activation achieved during a single repetition of weight training. Therefore, based on these discoveries, technically a single isometric exercise performed at only two-thirds of an individual's overall maximum can deliver either similar or often even better results, than the equivalent of up to 3 sets of 10 weight training repetitions in the lifting phase of the exercise.

To explain this further I will use a typical barbell curl exercise in the lifting phase as my example, where the object of the exercise is to engage as many muscle fibres as possible in a maximum muscular contraction. Naturally, 3 sets of 10 repetitions give us an overall total of 30 repetitions. One set of 10 repetitions of the barbell curl in perfect high-intensity style produces a total maximum muscular engagement for a total of approximately 3.3 seconds. Three sets of 10 repetitions of the same exercise, a total of 30 repetitions will give a total of approximately 9.9 seconds of maximum muscular engagement, and an average of 89% muscle activation overall.

In comparison, one high-intensity isometric contraction exercise produces a maximum muscular engagement that lasts for the entire duration of the exercise. Even though the optimum time over which an isometric exercise is performed was found to be 7 seconds, this is almost always rounded up to the 10-second target number. The maximum muscular engagement will last for the entire 10 seconds of a high-intensity isometric exercise and with 95.2% muscle activation overall.

This is proof that is based entirely on scientific research that 3 sets of 10 near-perfect high-intensity curls when weight training, which takes several minutes to perform, were still not equal to the results achieved by a single 10-second high-intensity isometric curl exercise.

The Standard Isometric Contraction

The standard isometric contraction is a simple and highly effective technique. Therefore, this is the technique we will focus on for practical isometric training. The standard isometric contraction, AKA: overcoming isometric contraction, AKA: maximum-effort isometrics, or whatever else you wish to call it, is when a muscle is applying force to push or pull against an immovable resistance. This is the most basic of all kinds of isometric exercise, and it is highly effective. This type of isometric contraction exercise was performed during the experiments by Dr T. Hettinger and Dr E. Muller at the Max Plank Institute. It is also the technique referred to in their book "The Physiology of Strength". In a standard isometric contraction, it is theoretically possible to exert up to 100% of one's maximum capacity effort against an immovable object and then continue to hold that level of force throughout the exercise. This means that standard isometric contraction can be a very high-intensity exercise system.

Performing an isometric exercise against an immovable object at a certain level of force for a given duration of time will teach your body to recruit more muscle fibres to try to move the object. As you perform the exercise and generate as much force as possible, your CNS, or Central Nervous System, learns that it needs to activate and recruit more muscle fibres to reach the goal of moving the object.

Since this will naturally be impossible to move, the process will continue each time you exercise to make you stronger and grow more muscle. Your body mechanisms become trained to readily activate and recruit additional muscle fibres as needed when facing repeated similar challenges, which in turn, repeats the cycle more readily every time.

As we mentioned earlier, the immovable/solid object that is used can be anything that is completely solid and completely safe to use. This can be a wall, a door, a door jamb, a parked motor vehicle, or anything similar. Perhaps the most common objects used to enhance everyday isometric exercise training are sturdy towels, climbing ropes, martial arts belts, scuba diving weight belts, webbing straps, golf clubs, and broom handles, etc. All the aforementioned items are excellent when used properly, and all will deliver some excellent results. More importantly, they are typically readily available for most people which makes exercising with them so much easier.

      Another common way to perform isometric exercise is to do it in a self-resisted way. Self-resisted means that you push or pull against your limbs, hands, and feet, etc. For example, you might place the palms of your hands together at chest level with your hands roughly at the midpoint of your body. In that position, press your hands together using your chest muscles to provide the primary driving force. Suddenly, you are performing a highly effective self-resisted isometric chest exercise!

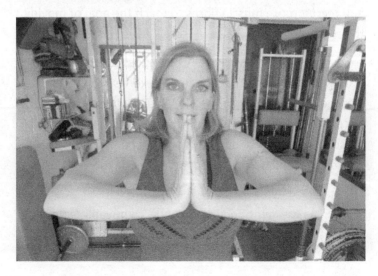

It is possible to perform a well-balanced and highly effective self-resisted isometric workout to exercise virtually every section of the body. So, never underestimate self-resisted exercise because it can be immensely powerful indeed. Also, self-resistance exercises are an excellent way to ensure that a personal maximum resistance is used safely, and with minimum risk of injury caused by applying too much force.

The fact is that it does not matter which method is chosen. It can be isometrics performed against an immovable object, self-resisted isometrics, or a combination of the two. The most important thing is that either the object must be completely immovable through human muscle power alone, or the force of one body part must be able to completely counterbalance the force of another body part to produce a muscular stalemate.

Workout Intensity

Intensity is always going to be a relative term, and it is often completely misunderstood when it is used concerning exercise. When it comes to exercising your muscles, the intensity is the % of your ability to move a resistance. Technically, an individual's highest possible level of intensity is when they reach a point of momentary failure after exerting themselves completely.

However, the important questions we need to try and find answers to are: "How hard is hard?" and "How intense is intense?" To some degree, both are very subjective things. Taking two people of roughly equal fitness, something that is intense to one person might be considered comparatively easy to the other. Hard is a relative term, and handling 50 lbs of resistance is impossibly hard if your strength is only at the level required to lift 49 lbs. However, if you can lift 100 lbs as a maximum, then lifting 50 lbs is going to be comparatively easy.

Often, the only factors differentiating between people and the intensity level exerted, are going to be mental toughness, determination, and perception. Therefore, to gain the greatest benefits from isometric exercise the first thing that must be learned is how to determine, with a reasonable degree of accuracy, what level of intensity is being applied to an exercise.

It is just a fact that what one person deems to be 100% of their capacity will always be quite different from another person's estimate. The accurate estimation of what one person deems to be 2/3^{rds} of their overall maximum force and intensity will also vary from person to person. The accuracy of estimation will also vary greatly between an experienced professional athlete and an absolute beginner to exercise.

Experience has taught us that most people who are new to exercise will always fall well short of accurate estimation of any given percentage. A beginner will find it more challenging to accurately estimate what 2/3^{rds} of their 100% maximum is when compared to a more experienced athlete. Many people might believe that they are performing at 100% capacity when they are only performing at around 2/3^{rds}, or even perhaps at only 50% or less of their 100% maximum. This is because exercise is new to them, therefore, the experiences and feelings in their body which are associated with it are also new. They simply have no common frame of reference when it comes to calculating/estimating their level of physical exertion.

The human brain has a built-in mechanism that helps to protect the body and prevent it from performing a physical activity to such a level that could cause serious damage or even death. This is the mechanism that makes your brain tell you to stop exercising when it begins to get tough, and the feeling of wanting to stop exercising only increases as you continue to push yourself harder to do more. This is all despite the biological fact that you are physically capable of doing much more than is being suggested by the messages you are receiving from yourself.

Over time, the brain of people who exercise regularly, and especially to a high level of intensity, will naturally adjust, and reposition this built-in safety margin. This means that the brain of an experienced high-level athlete does not "tell" them to stop an exercise until the level of intensity is much higher than it would be for a beginner. Therefore, when it comes to exercise, how is it possible to subjectively quantify, and then impart appropriate levels of recommended intensity? This problem is made even more challenging when one considers the fact that accurately translating and subjectively assessing various levels of intensity will, to some degree, always be subjective to every individual.

If you were to train as hard as humanly possible, with near 100% maximum intensity which involves super-strict form, and training to complete failure and beyond, then you simply cannot train for a long time. It is just physiologically impossible. Physics and biology are quite simple in this respect. The intensity of your workout is directly proportional to the length of time that you are physically able to perform your workout. The harder and more intensely you exercise, the shorter time that you will be physically able to perform the exercise.

Make no mistake, performing a 7-second isometric exercise while exerting close to your personal 100% maximum physical capacity is completely and utterly exhausting, even for a professional athlete. What does all this mean when it comes to accurately communicating various levels of exercise force and intensity, especially when there is no professional coach or elaborate and expensive measuring equipment at hand?

Research clearly shows that almost everyone will stop exercising long before they are in any danger of becoming seriously fatigued. Most people will *think* they are achieving a much higher level of intensity than they would if they were only a little more mentally resilient. This does not mean that people should suddenly begin pushing themselves beyond their physical limits, which would be a stupid thing to do. However, it does mean that most people who enjoy a higher-than-average level of mental resilience and determination, as well as being in physically good condition, can push themselves much harder than they might think. If anyone ever feels "genuine" strain or fatigue to the point of becoming injured, then they should stop exercising immediately.

Even without the aid of a professional coach to monitor, encourage you and measure your intensity and progress with specialist equipment, the tips we have outlined in this section will help you to get the most out of every workout. It is also worth remembering that if you cheat, then the only person who loses is "you."

As a footnote, for the sake of clarification. Exercise intensity refers to how much energy is expended when exercising which includes the amount of weight used per repetition, and Perceived intensity varies with each person. Intensity and force are technically different but are frequently accepted as interchangeable terms in the common vernacular. Muscular strength is different from muscular endurance, which is the ability to produce and sustain muscle force over a certain period of time. While strength is the maximum force you can apply against a load, power is proportional to the speed at which you can explosively apply it. In other words, it is the ability to produce a given amount of force quickly. Muscular force, often referred to as muscular strength, is the physical power exerted by muscles to perform various actions, such as lifting, pushing, or pulling objects. It results from the contraction of muscles and is vital for human mobility and functionality.

Technically, How Does a Muscle Grow?

How does a muscle grow? This is one of the most common questions asked concerning fitness and exercise in general. However, it is also one of the most misunderstood concepts, even amongst fitness professionals and personal trainers. To see for yourself just how uninformed or badly informed some people are, simply join one or two of the social media groups online so you can read some of the absolute drivel posted by 'keyboard warriors' who purport to be 'experts' on the subject. Alarmingly, many of these people seem to have developed a hardcore following, which to the science-based professional is like watching 'fools leading other fools' on a wild goose chase.

So, back to the key question which is, how does a muscle grow? To explain this, we must examine three concepts, which are: 1) muscle growth through increases in the volume/size of myofibrils inside the muscles, which is commonly called myofibrillar hypertrophy. 2) hyperplasia, which is when there is an increase in the number of muscle cells/fibres. 3) sarcoplasmic growth which is all about increasing the fluid content.

When it comes to the subject of exercise, the muscles you wish to grow must be challenged with a workload that is greater than they can currently accommodate. In other words, an exercise that is intense enough to stimulate growth. This stimulus can come from any source such as lifting a heavy object, weight training, isometrics, compressing a spring in a device such as a Bullworker™, or through self-resistance either hand to hand or limb to limb or using an Iso-Bow™ etc.

This process creates trauma to the muscle fibres which disrupts the muscle cell organelles. This then triggers other cells outside the muscle fibres to greatly increase in numbers at and around the point of the trauma to repair the damage. The process of repair involves a fusion of cells. This, in turn, causes the cross-sectional area of the muscle fibre to increase because the muscle cell myofibrils increase in both size and quantity. This process is more commonly known as hypertrophy. Since this process increases the number of cellular nuclei the muscle fibres generate more myosin and actin. These are contractile protein myofilaments which in turn help to make the muscle stronger.

This is the basis of what is more commonly known as myofibril muscle growth. In addition to this, there is also probably a process called hyperplasia which takes place. I use the term, 'probably' because this concept is extremely controversial for many reasons. One of the key problems is that evidence of this in human beings is lacking, whereas there is a mass of evidence supporting hyperplasia in mice and other animals.

Hypertrophy is the increase in the size of the existing muscle fibres to accommodate the increased demands placed upon them through intense exercise. Hyperplasia, concerning skeletal muscle growth, is the increase in the number of muscle fibres which in turn will also increase the cross-sectional area of a muscle.

Despite there being a lack of evidence supporting hyperplasia in human beings, logic supports the process taking place. This is because of a theory known as Nuclear Domain Theory. This states that the nucleus of a cell (a muscle cell in this instance) is only able to control a finite area of cellular space. It is thought that satellite cells donate their nuclei to the muscle cell until a certain point is reached whereby this can no longer take place. Beyond a certain limit, and through continued intense training, the cell must eventually divide to create two cells instead of the former single cell. When this happens, the entire hypertrophy process starts over once again. This probably means that most of the muscle growth is almost certainly caused by hypertrophy, and a much smaller percentage can be attributed to hyperplasia at any given point in the muscle stimulus/growth process.

Finally, there is a subject of sarcoplasmic muscle growth to address. Sarcoplasmic muscle growth is the increase in the volume of sarcoplasmic fluid in the muscle cell. These are the fluid and energy resources surrounding the myofibrils in your muscles containing mostly glycogen together with other elements including creatine, ATP, and water etc.

To clarify, glycogen is simply a type of sugar that serves as a form of energy. It is deposited in bodily tissues as a store of carbohydrates, and it is the body's main form of storage for the sugar, glucose. Glycogen is stored in two main places in the body, one being the liver, and the other being the muscles.

More importantly, glycogen is the body's secondary source of long-term energy storage, with the primary energy storage source being fat. When glycogen is in the muscles, it is converted into glucose for use as energy when performing sports etc., and glycogen stored in the liver is converted into glucose for use as energy throughout the body, and in the central nervous system.

Therefore, sarcoplasmic growth increases muscle volume, but this increase is not in functional strength mass since it does not increase the number of muscle fibres. It is like 'the pump', in that it is an increase in the size and shape of the muscle through the muscle holding an increased amount of fluid.

Rest Time Between Exercises

Naturally, the rest time taken between exercises during a workout is quite different from the rest and recovery needed to recover and allow your body to positively respond to the stimulus generated by exercise.

If you keep the rest time between exercises brief enough, then the workout routine itself will give you an excellent cardiovascular workout, and this is what we recommend that you ultimately aim for. If you are already very fit, then we would recommend that instead of performing the optional cardio routine, you simply put more effort, force, and overall intensity into each isometric exercise. At the same time, aim to keep the rest time between those exercises as brief as possible. This approach will help you work towards being able to perform each exercise so that it has an Ultra-High Intensity Ultra-Short Burst™ effect, which will greatly improve your overall fitness level, and boost your Base Metabolic Rate or BMR.

However, if you are not already fit, then to begin with you may wish to simply allow each isometric exercise to deliver all the cardio you need as you gradually build up your levels of fitness and endurance. Eventually, you will increase your level of fitness to a point where you can begin to gradually reduce the rest time between each exercise to a minimum point that works best for you.

Once you have learned how to fully engage the muscles during each exercise with sufficient force, and at the same time, you have learned how to breathe fully, deeply, and naturally throughout each exercise. At the same time, you should be keeping the rest time between exercises to a minimum because this combination will have an excellent and beneficial cardiovascular effect.

Dynamic Flexation™

Dynamic Flexation™ is a technique we devised to help ensure that we gained maximum benefit from the isometric portion of our exercise regimens. I will recap and briefly summarise the Dynamic Flexation™ technique as originally laid out in "The 70 Second Difference™" book.

We always recommend that everyone who performs any kind of resistance exercise practices some form of Dynamic Flexation™ before performing any exercise. This will help to ensure that all muscles, tendons, ligaments, joints, and your spine have become naturally and properly engaged in the correct biomechanical exercise position.

We would never recommend that as soon as you assume any exercise position you suddenly apply maximum power and force right away. This is unless you are a very experienced athlete, or unless you are training with a qualified coach to perform a certain type of isometric exercise to develop extra power such as a static-dynamic or explosive/ballistic isometric technique. Instead, we recommend that you always breathe naturally as you gradually flex and engage your muscles and joints into performing the exercise.

To perform Dynamic Flexation™ you gradually flex your grip and the muscles you are about to exercise while applying an increasing level of force immediately before performing the exercise. The exercise is then performed, and to disengage from the exercise we recommend reversing the Dynamic Flexation™ engagement process.

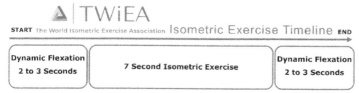

Our preference is to apply tension and force to the exercise gradually through Dynamic Flexation™ typically for between 2 and 3 seconds, or even for as long as 4 seconds if needed. This all takes place before beginning to count the required 7-second exercise time of the isometric contraction. We prefer using one deep full breath in and out as a method of more accurately counting each second that has elapsed. This way, you will time each exercise more accurately, and you will not be tempted to hold your breath at any point which is a mistake that beginners often make. Similarly, at the end of an exercise, we do not recommend that it be ended abruptly. Instead, we recommend reversing the Dynamic Flexation™ technique so that you gradually relax as you slightly move each muscle and joint out of the exercise position.

This process helps enormously because when you are in a good position it will help you to gain the maximum benefit from each exercise you perform. Dynamic Flexation™ is when you move and adjust your feet, legs, hips and especially your hands as you gradually assume a solid position and handgrip. As you flex and move, you will be making micro-adjustments.

All exercises will be performed best if you assume a correct and solid handgrip, fist clench, or foot position etc.

One of the most important aspects of assuming the correct exercise position begins with your grip. Without a solid grip on a bar, handle, or anything else you need to hold while exercising, you will naturally be setting yourself up to perform sub-maximally. You can also be helping to develop injuries which can include sore elbows, joints, ligaments, and tendons.

Dynamic Flexation™ is a concept that embraces the broader principles of motor unit recruitment, and "Henneman's Size Principle" to increase the contractile strength of a muscle. Elwood Henneman's principle stated that under load, the motor units in a muscle are engaged according to their magnitude of force output, from the smallest to the largest, and in task-appropriate order. This means that the slow-twitch, low-force, fatigue-resistant muscle fibres are activated before any fast-twitch, high-force muscle fibres are engaged which are less fatigue-resistant. Since the body naturally works in this way, it enables precise and finely controlled force to be delivered at all levels of output. This also means that when exercising, or when performing tasks in daily life, the fatigue which is experienced as a result will always be minimised. It will also be proportional to the sequential engagement of the most appropriate muscle fibres being engaged.

Isometric Exercises and Blood Pressure

Some exercise critics point out the fact that when someone performs an isometric exercise it will raise their blood pressure. However, the same people also very conveniently forget that the same is also true of all other forms of exercise including freehand callisthenics and traditional isotonic resistance training with weights. ALL physical activity, and especially exercise will cause your blood pressure to rise for a short time. Providing that you are in good health, and you always breathe deeply, naturally, and normally when performing any exercise, any rise in blood pressure will soon return to a normal level when the exercise is stopped. The faster this happens, the fitter you are.

For those who are advanced athletes and/or are used to hard and intense isometric training for a long time, you will already have made significant progress in strengthening your heart and circulatory system. For those who are new to isometric training, just like with any form of exercise, the best way into it is by taking it slowly and less intensely at first. Newcomers to exercise, and especially isometrics, should always focus on applying less force and overall intensity, to begin with, and on always breathing fully and deeply throughout all exercises. NEVER HOLD YOUR BREATH! Under strict medical supervision, even those with Coronary Artery Disease and high blood pressure should be able to increase their physical activity levels with a reasonable degree of safety. However, if you are a person who already suffers from high blood pressure, then you should always exercise at a much lower level of force and overall intensity than someone who has no physical issues.

Furthermore, **EVERYONE, ESPECIALLY PEOPLE WITH HYPERTENSION, OR ANY FORM OF CARDIOVASCULAR DISEASE, SHOULD ALWAYS CHECK WITH THEIR DOCTOR BEFORE BEGINNING ANY KIND OF EXERCISE ROUTINE.**

Rest and Recovery

When calculating your ideal recovery period, many things must be taken into consideration. These include your age, your current health and fitness level, the quantity of exercise taken, and most importantly the intensity of the exercise which has been performed.

Some people will need a recovery period of between 24 and 48 hours, and for others, the recovery period may be as brief as between 12 and 24 hours.

As a rule, the recovery period will always incrementally increase as the intensity of the exercises increases towards an individual's 100% potential maximum capacity. Always be aware of this and make sure that you factor this into your rest and recovery time calculations. The diagram will help to outline this.

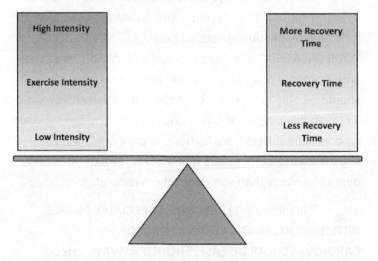

Sports scientist J. Atha's research revealed something remarkable. This was that when performing isometric contraction exercises at two-thirds of an individual's maximum capacity, the average person could safely perform an exercise like this daily, without overtraining.

Standard isometric contraction exercises can be safely performed daily, by almost anyone, of almost any age, and in almost any physical condition as a means of strength development, body shaping, and even bodybuilding. However, for more intense workouts, we recommend a full rest day between workouts due to the higher demands being placed upon the Central Nervous System (CNS) and the time needed to fully recover and benefit from the exercise.

Several other factors affect post-exercise recovery. These include a balanced and properly executed stretching routine and getting enough quality sleep. While you sleep, your body releases certain hormones which help you to repair and rebuild damaged tissue, and which will directly help your muscles to grow.

Adequate Nutrition is Vital

Quality post-exercise nutrition will help your body repair itself faster, decrease your recovery time, and help to maximise the benefits gained from the exercise. Research shows that post-exercise immunodepression peaks if you exercise for longer than you are currently capable, and problems are enhanced due to reduced or inadequate nutrition. Hydration is also one of the most important factors in your recovery, as well as for your overall health, especially since your muscles are mostly composed of water.

Early studies suggested a 30 to 60-minute window after exercise when you need to eat, after which, your body begins to draw upon itself to repair and recover from your workout. Later studies found that this window can be anything from 1 to 3 hours depending on the workout type, applied force, overall intensity, and goals. On average, since most leave 60 minutes after food before hard exercise, and if a workout lasts an average of 45 minutes, then a 30 to 45-minute window to eat after exercise will mean it has been up to 150 minutes (2.5 hours) since your last food, therefore, the earlier suggested 30–45-minute window still makes sense for most people especially if they want to build more muscle and strength.

Most people mistakenly consume excessive amounts of protein at the expense of other key nutrients such as carbohydrates. Therefore, in doing this they are working against their best interests and overall optimum health. One of the key nutrients that have been found to help enormously when in recovery from prolonged periods of heavy exercise is carbohydrates. A lot of research supports the hypothesis that carbohydrate is the most important nutritional factor in preventing post-exercise immunodepression. Most do not realise that the protein composition of human muscle is typically only somewhere in the region of between 18/9% and 21% protein (average 20%) and the rest is made up of water, glucose, lipids, and carbohydrates etc. We will not go into more detail here, however, if you want to learn more about this and many other surprising nuggets of useful information about sensible nutrition and exercise then they can be found in The 70 Second Difference book.

Strength, Stamina, Endurance, and Resilience

It is important to understand the difference between strength, stamina and endurance because once understood, you will then be able to devise the most suitable workout routines according to your body type.

Muscular strength is possibly best understood as being a muscle's capacity to exert force against resistance, or weight. This is comparatively easy to measure because your ability to lift a given amount of weight for a single repetition is a good measure of your strength.

Stamina is the length of time at which a muscle, or group of muscles, can perform at or near its maximum capacity. For example, the number of squats you can perform with a given weight which is 90% of your maximum would be a measure of your stamina or the distance which you can carry a similarly heavy object such as an anvil.

Endurance is all about time, and your ability to perform a certain muscular action for a prolonged period regardless of the capacity at which you are working.

Resilience is all about your ability to recover from whatever stresses and demands are placed on your muscles. However, resilience is mostly all about your state of mind, your mental toughness and ability to endure, perform and deliver under pressure, and how you recover quickly emotionally.

The muscular composition of your body will always determine how well you will perform in certain sports. The amount of slow twitch muscle fibres you possess will determine how well you perform at endurance-related events, and both type A and type B fast twitch muscle fibres are all about explosive power and your ability to maintain it. In simple terms, if you possess mostly slow twitch fibres, then you are naturally going to be better suited to endurance sports. Alternatively, if you possess mostly fast twitch muscle fibres, then you are a natural weightlifter. It is important to note, that no matter what your natural predisposition might be in this respect, with the correct training regimen, it is still possible to significantly increase your abilities in your naturally weaker opposing areas of speciality.

Biceps, Supination, and Strong Arms

When most people think about the biceps muscles, they only think about flexing the biceps and elbow joints to create a classic bodybuilder pose. However, there is a great deal more to the biceps muscles than this. While flexing the arm in the way I have just described might be a primary function, another equally primary function is the action of twisting the forearm and hand, otherwise known as supination. This is it in pictures.

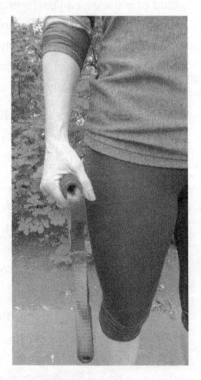

Neutral Position Front

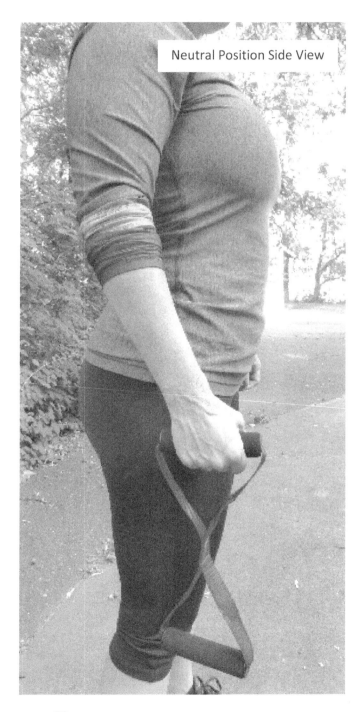

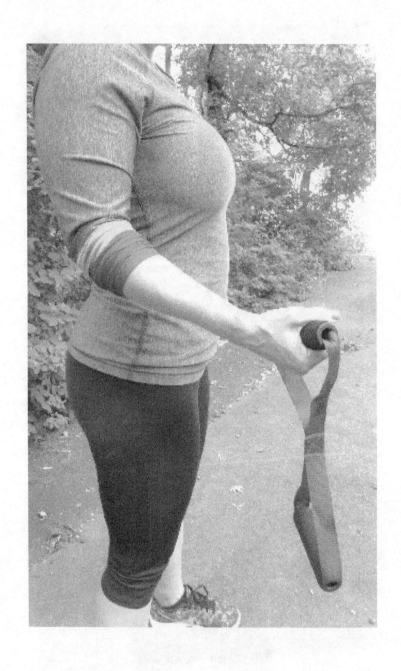

Mid Supination Side View

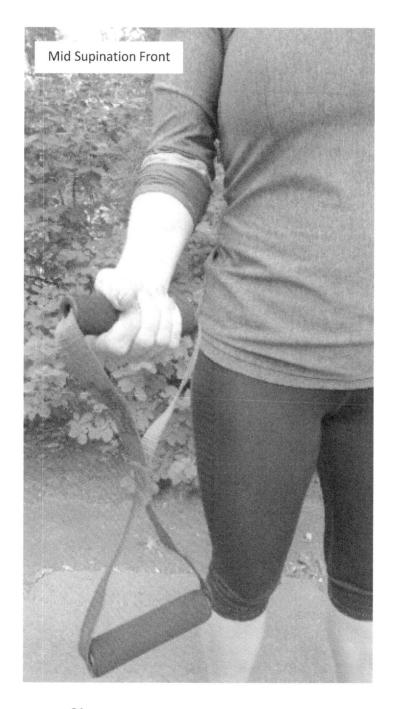

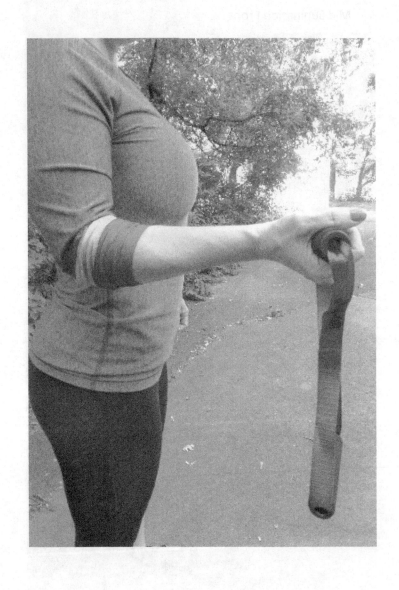

Full Supination Side

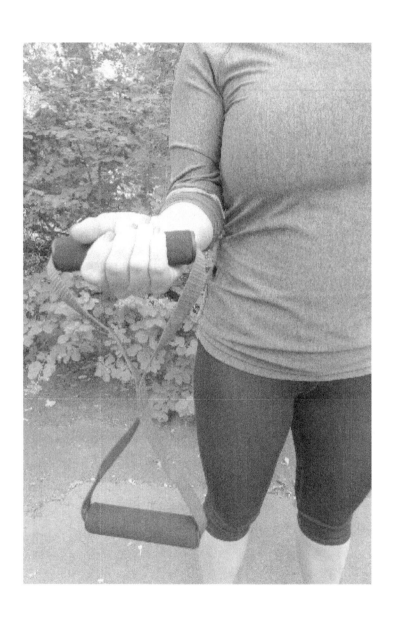

Full Supination Front View

Supination starts with the hand in a neutral position, roughly parallel to the side of your upper thigh, and twisting it as it is being raised until your palm is facing upwards at the top of the movement when the biceps are fully flexed.

The brachialis muscle is the primary mover of elbow flexion and not the biceps brachii as most people think. This is because, even though the biceps brachii "show" muscle is seen flexed during a classic biceps pose, it is the brachialis that underlies it that generates about 50% more power than the biceps brachii.

Therefore, supination is not only important to elbow rotation but overall upper arm strength. Therefore, to gain maximum benefit and strength when exercising your overall front upper arm, all component muscles and their actions must be taken into consideration.

The problem with isometric exercise in this respect when pitting one limb against another limb, or static immovable objects such as a wall, door or chair is that it does not naturally allow the brachialis muscle to be exercised effectively.

This is where the iso-Bow® fills the gap and enables a range of exercises to be performed in a neutral, partial, or fully supinated position.

Chapter 4: All Things Iso-Bow®

A common question we are asked is: "Is it necessary to use the Iso-Bow® to perform an effective isometric or self-resisted workout?" This is a good question.

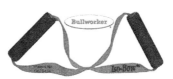

No, it is not necessary to use an Iso-Bow®, but we believe that it is better if you do, and there are several reasons why.

Firstly, it is all about the science and safety of biomechanics. A stable line of biomechanical progression all begins with a correctly positioned grip, a firm grip, and the progression in continuing that stability through correctly aligned joints and limbs while you perform the exercise.

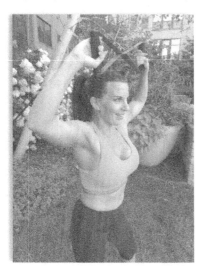

The same is true in isometric exercise because it all begins with a stable line of biomechanical progression. This starts with either a properly clenched hand or fist and continues that stability through correctly aligned joints and limbs to perform the isometric hold.

This is just one reason why we fully recommend and endorse the Iso-Bow® because it makes this whole process much easier. It has a well-designed and comfortable non-slip handgrip, which allows you to execute a firm, stable handgrip position to begin creating a stable line of biomechanical progression.

The Iso-Bow® is a product we fully endorse and highly recommend. It is inexpensive, high quality, and it

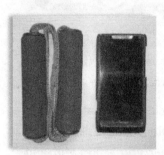

works exceptionally well. An amazing Iso-Bow® costs "pennies" in comparison to other exercise devices, and even a pair of them can easily fit into your pocket, they never need adjusting, and they can deliver a total-body workout at the perfect level of intensity for either a completely unfit beginner or an advanced athlete!

If you have already read "The 70 Second Difference™" book, then you will also know that we are not even endorsing our product. We are simply endorsing a product which we believe will be the best investment you

will ever make if you want to get fit, strong, and in the best shape of your life. The company that makes the Iso-Bow® is Hughes Marketing LLC,

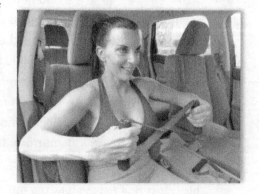

and they also produce a small range of other highly effective exercise products, which all deliver excellent results at a fair price.

The Iso-Bow® is versatile too, and it can be used with equal effectiveness as both an isotonic and an isometric exercise device. It allows the user to perform highly effective self-resisted isotonic exercises for almost every muscle group.

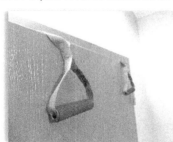

A pair of Iso-Bows® can even be used as a great doorway pull-up device, which can even fold up and slip right into your pocket when you are done. Try doing that with a regular, clumsy steel doorway pull-up bar!

The Iso-Bow® is naturally a first-class isometric exercise device, and it allows a very wide range of exercises to be performed that work almost every muscle

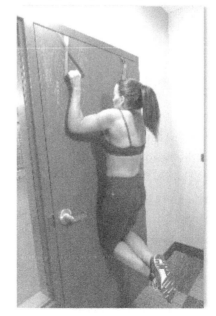

group of the body. It also allows the effective execution of more advanced techniques to be performed within the ISOfitness™ system.

Since the Iso-Bow® is so inexpensive, well-designed, well-constructed, and extremely useful in ways we haven't even begun to describe here in this book, it is not so much a recommendation for you to get a pair, but rather an instruction for you to do so. We believe that you will soon see why these inexpensive devices are what we believe to be the finest, most versatile, and most powerful of all exercise devices which have ever been invented!

That is a bold statement, but it is made because of our sincere belief in the product, and how you will benefit from owning a pair if you use them correctly. Do not forget, that we do not make this product, we simply believe in it to that degree of commitment.

Securing the Iso-Bow® With Your Feet

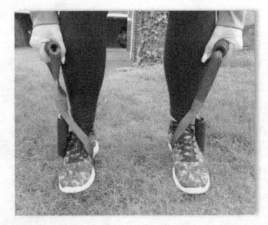

When performing leg exercises such as squats and lunges, as well as lower back and glute exercises such as the deadlift, it becomes necessary to properly secure the Iso-Bow® using your feet.

There are several ways in which the Iso-Bow® can be secured using your feet, and your personal preference of how you do this will depend upon many factors such

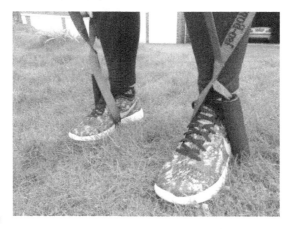

as your foot size, your choice of footwear, and ease of operation.

You can secure the Iso-Bow® with your foot inside one of the handles. You do this by adjusting the handgrip to

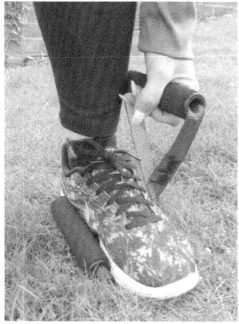

one side, usually the outer side of the foot, and then placing your feet inside the loop like a stirrup.

Another method is to place the Iso-Bow® flat on the floor and then stand on one side of the straps so that the handle of the same side sits flush with your inner foot. In this position, it will be your bodyweight combined with the handle pressing against the inner side of your foot which 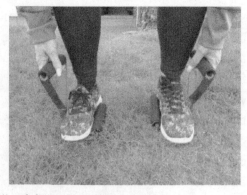 enables you to pull safely and securely.

The final method is to simply place each foot 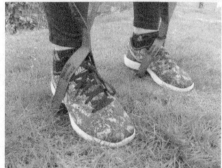 through one end of an Iso-Bow®, stepping onto the foam handgrip as you do so. This method is slightly less stable than the other two methods. However, if the foot can be pushed far enough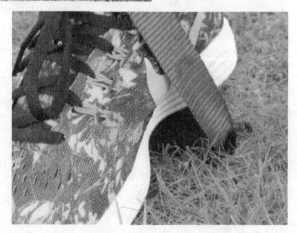

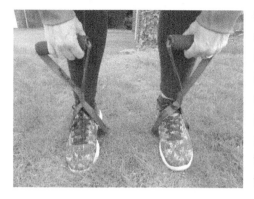 through the loop of the Iso-Bow® handle, then the handle will slightly raise the level of your heel making it easier for some people to squat or lunge.

Naturally, safety is always a top priority so whichever method you ultimately choose to use, you should always make sure that when securing the Iso-Bow® with your feet there is never any chance of it slipping in any way while you exercise.

Shortening The Iso-Bow® - The Cradle

Generally, the Iso-Bow® is the ideal size for most people to use with each exercise. However, occasionally you may prefer to reduce its operational size by roughly half, by creating what we call an Iso-Bow® cradle.

To do this you place one of the handles inside the webbing loop of the other handle side of the device. The handle you have just placed inside the loop is then cradled by the webbing and can be gripped as normal. Your thumb and fingers can then wrap around both the foam handle and the webbing of the cradle loop to help ensure an even firmer grip position is created.

This reduced size allows for an even greater operational range within the movement capability of each limb/joint to be created for certain exercises. These include

The Cross-Chest Press, the Upper Back Power Pull, and the Biceps and Triceps Cradle Press-Curl.

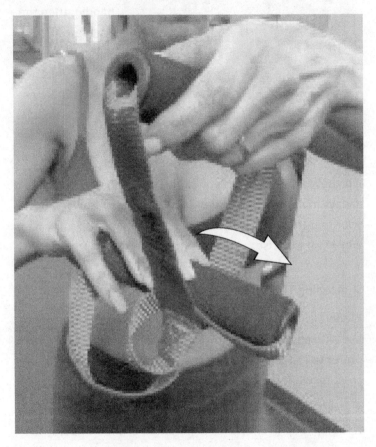

Chapter 5: About the Exercise Model

Helen Renée is an American who is married to a Brit. She was born in Minnesota and grew up in Northern Alaska after her father became an Ice Road Trucker.

Helen went from being 40 lbs overweight to a contest-winning condition almost effortlessly in less than 6 months and with workout sessions lasting no longer than 10 minutes per day.

Helen is an isometric exercise expert instructor and champion Bikini Fitness Athlete who achieved spectacular contest-winning results after meeting her exercise scientist husband.

Helen's husband is one of the world's leading experts on isometric exercise, plant-based nutrition, and was a former coach to the 4-times World's Strongest Man, Jon Pall Sigmarsson of Iceland.

Currently, Helen has co-authored 21 fitness books and since she and her husband share a common fascination with mysteries and the paranormal, they have co-authored a best-selling book on the subject.

Since meeting and marrying her British husband they have enjoyed a joyous journey together discovering the many differences between the two countries which share a common language and culture.

They began writing these stories and anecdotes down and very soon had enough to produce a fun-filled and light-hearted book about what it is like Being American Married to a Brit.

Helen is remarkably strong with the exceptional power-to-weight ratio one would expect from a former gymnast.

She is also an isometric and TRISOmetric™ exercise instructor, consultant, and instructor-trainer for TWiEA™ The World Isometric Exercise Association. www.TWiEA.com – www.HelenRenee.com

The following pictures are of Helen Renée taken in January 2015 before she started performing a daily 10 x 7-second total-body exercise isometric exercise routine.

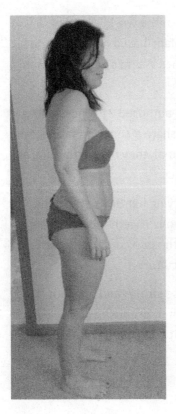
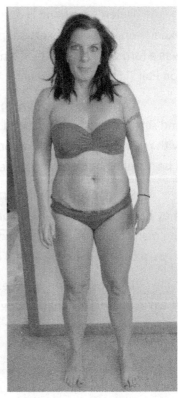

The following pictures are of Helen Renée 1-year later, in January 2016. She became a contest-winning Bikini Fitness competitor within 1-year of daily isometric exercise training lasting only minutes each day. Now, Helen trains using only isometric exercises because they are so effective and time-efficient. She simply exercises regularly each day and applies more force and overall intensity to each exercise than a normal person who simply wants to get a little stronger, fitter and maintain a good overall body shape. Helen also eats sensibly.

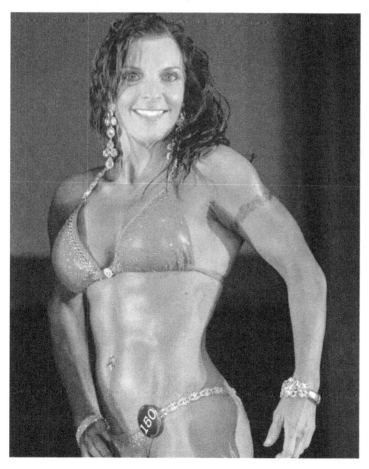

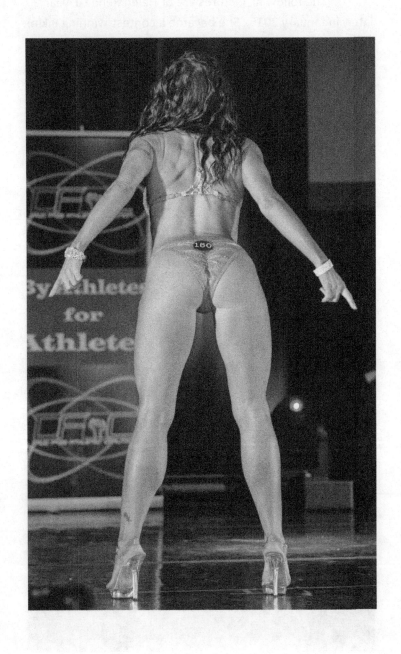

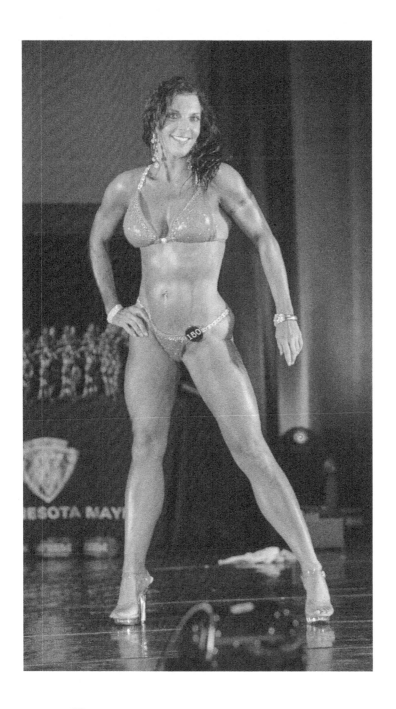

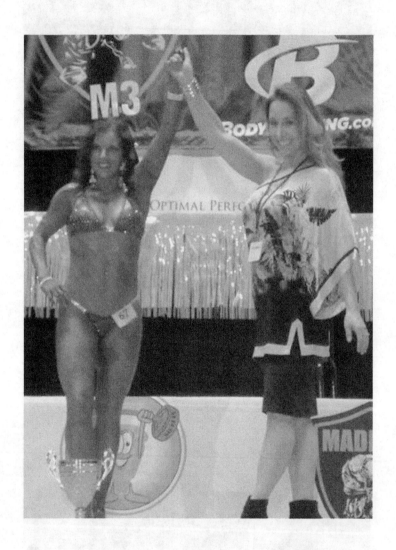

The Author and an Isometric Experiment

The following picture is of my arm taken in December 2016. This was the result of a year-long experiment to see what results could be gained through a basic high-intensity isometric exercise routine using only the minimum number of exercises.

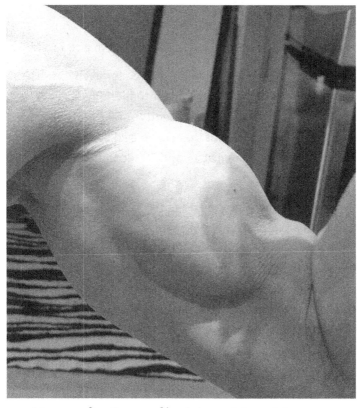

My arm after 1 year of basic isometric maintenance training. This picture was taken to record the results of the experiment in December 2016.
The routine allowed just 1 x 7-second isometric exercise per muscle/muscle group per day at a target level of applied force/intensity of between 75% and 80%.

For one year, starting in January 2016, I performed a daily 10-exercise x 7-second total-body isometric routine. It is common for even the most experienced athletes to count the elapsed exercise time increasingly quickly, almost in direct proportion to an increasing level of applied force/intensity.

Therefore, I typically aimed to perform a 10-second isometric hold for each exercise, and this way I would always reach the desired goal of 7 seconds in good style.

My target level of applied force for each exercise was around 75-80%, slightly higher than the typically recommended average of two-thirds or 66.6%. However, this still effectively meant that I exercised each of my biceps for a total of between just 21 and 30 seconds per week, nothing more.

Amazingly, at the end of the year-long experiment, I achieved an improvement in both the strength and size of each arm, albeit slightly. Even though I am well-versed in the science of isometrics I still found it remarkable because it was in exchange for a maximum of 30 seconds per week of exercise time. Once again, this only served to reinforce the fact that the best results are always gained through pinpoint focus, applied force, overall high intensity, and never confusing activity with accomplishment.

Chapter 6: Things to Remember Before You Begin

- The first and perhaps the most important thing to remember is: **NEVER HOLD YOUR BREATH AT ANY TIME.**
- Breathing in and out naturally during all isometric exercises will also help you count the number of elapsed seconds much more accurately, with one full breath in and out taking approximately one second.
- We recommend that you read the instructions about each exercise carefully. You can also watch the associated videos via the TWiEA™ website if you wish to become a member and access the resource.
- Always leave a safe distance between you and others if exercising with any proprietary device or IIED (Improvised Isometric Exercise Device)
- Always check the structural integrity of any type of exercise device. If there is any doubt about the structural integrity, then do not use it for exercise or any other purpose.
- Double-check that any/all adjustable joints on the exercise device and/or IIED are secure before use.
- Weight loss/fat loss will ONLY occur when any exercise plan is used in conjunction with a calorie-controlled diet.
- It is critically important to completely focus your mind on the exercise being performed. Envision the muscle you are exercising growing larger and stronger.
- Always consult a professional coach to devise a detailed stretching routine, this will ensure that you

- are stretching the areas effectively rather than risking injury.
- Always ensure that a stable line of biomechanical progression is achieved before engaging in and performing any exercise.
- Warming-up, stretching, and cooling down are three of the most overlooked yet essential elements of exercise, and we cannot stress their importance strongly enough.
- During ANY form of physical exercise, including isometrics, if you apply too much force too soon, then you may inadvertently strain a muscle. Isometric exercise is particularly intense, and a single isometric exercise engages a great many more muscle fibres than even high-intensity weight training, and at a much higher level.

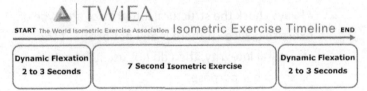

For safety's sake, we always recommend using Dynamic Flexation™ to engage your muscles gradually and progressively into ANY exercise, especially isometrics, according to what we call The ISOfitness Exercise Engagement Timeline™.

The main benefit of properly warming up for several minutes before a workout is injury prevention and increasing your heart rate and circulation to your muscles, ligaments, and tendons. It is important to remember that warming-up and stretching are two different concepts and that stretching is not a good warm-up. This is because stretching will put the muscle in an un-contracted position and weaken it. Stretching is always best performed after a workout has been completed, together with a proper cool-down.

In addition to properly warming-up, always perform a gentle flex and stretch of the muscles and joints which are about to be exercised. For example, squatting down fully to flex the thighs and loosen the knees is always a good idea before performing any leg exercises. Dynamic Flexation™ performed before any exercise should help to ensure greater flexibility and increased blood supply to the muscles and surrounding tissue.

Isometric exercises are deceptively powerful. Even when engaging in what may feel like only moderate-intensity exercise, you are probably still engaging and contracting many more muscle fibres than you would in a similar isotonic exercise. Therefore, if you are in any doubt whatsoever, then always perform the exercise with a little less force and overall intensity.

All exercises and workout plans work equally well for men and women. Both sexes can build strength, muscle, body build, or simply get into great shape if so desired, each according to their natural ability.

In our exercise resource books, the exercises listed are suggestions of what can be performed for each body part/muscle group. We are not suggesting that they should all be performed. Instead, users may wish to select the most suitable exercises from each section. In our course books, please perform the exercises according to the workout session notes.

Finally, please read, review, and ensure that you have fully complied with all recommendations in the section entitled: 'Important General Safety and Health Guidelines,' and only start using the isometric, or any exercise system with the full approval of your physician.

Chapter 7: Fitness on the Move™ Exercises
Abdominals: Knee Raise and Trunk Curl

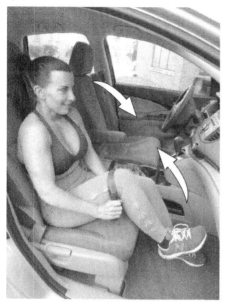

Sit on a seat, or any other solid object, and place the Iso-Bow® with handles facing downwards, over the top of one knee.

Then, curl your body forwards and downwards by contracting the abdominals, at the same time, raise the knee resisted by the Iso-Bow®.

Always breathe deeply and naturally as you perform the exercise, which will be about 10 full breaths, at a rate of about 1 second per breath.

Perform each exercise for no less than 7 seconds, and no longer than 10.

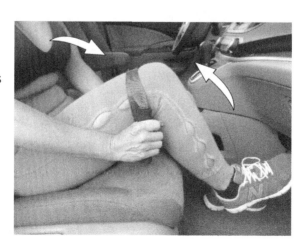

Repeat the exercise using the other knee.

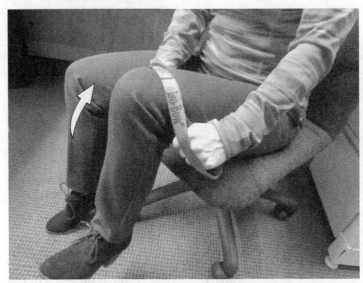

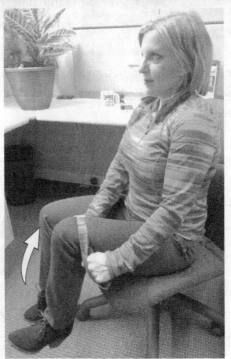

Alternative Exercise Without an Iso-Bow®

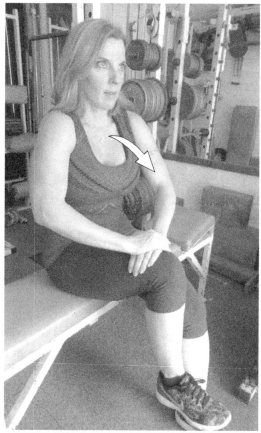

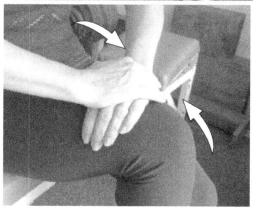

Iso-Bow® V-Sit Side-to-Side

Lay down and raise your legs and torso off the floor by curling the spine, at the same time gripping the Iso-Bow® securely with both hands close to your midsection.

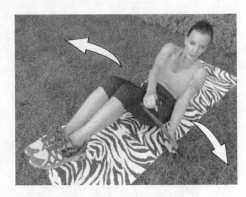

Twist the Iso-Bow® to one side as you engage the abdominal and oblique muscles.

Breathe naturally and deeply in and out for about 10 full breaths, which will take about 1 second per breath.

Aim to perform an exercise breathing count of no less than 7 seconds, and no longer than 10 seconds. Repeat the exercise on the other side of your body.

For additional resistance, perform a regular trunk curl with bent knees, while at the same time, resisting the motion with an Iso-Bow® wrapped across both knees as shown.

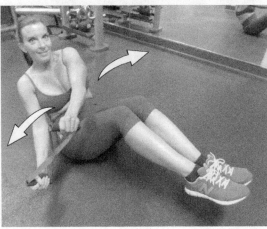

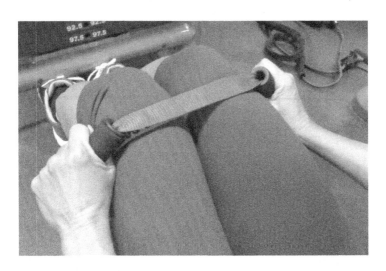

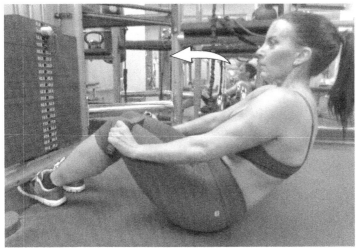

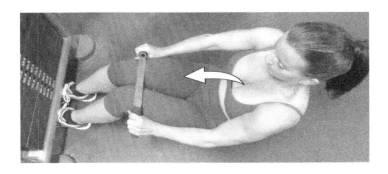

Alternative Exercise Without an Iso-Bow®

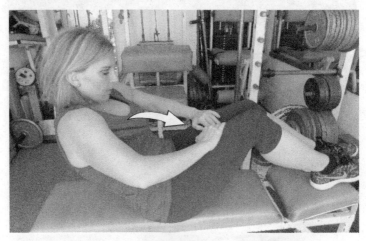

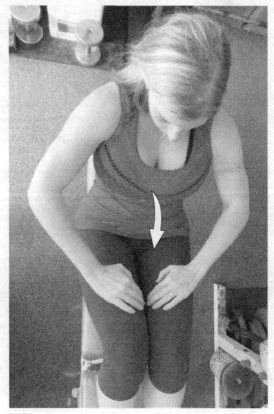

Iso-Bow® Kneeling Side Bend
(Iso-Bow® Loop Secured Under Each Knee)

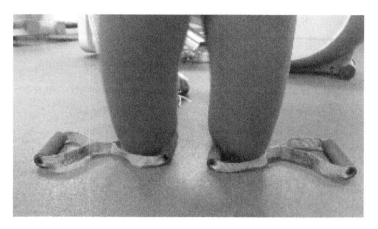

Kneel on the floor with your legs about shoulder-width apart and place the open loop of an Iso-Bow® comfortably under each knee so that the handle will be secured by your kneeling leg.

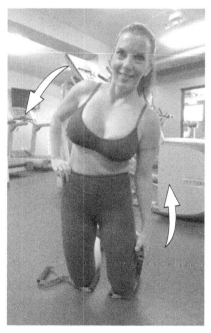

Keeping your hips upright and in the neutral position, bend sideways until you can hold one Iso-Bow® handle.

In that position, use your abdominal oblique muscles on the opposite side of your body to attempt to pull you in an upright direction. Naturally, you will not be able to move as you apply resistance and lock into an isometric exercise.

Repeat the exercise on the other side and be sure to never hold both Iso-Bow® handles at the same time.

Breathe naturally and deeply in and out for about 10 full breaths, which will take about 1 second per breath. Aim to perform an exercise breathing count of no less than 7 seconds, and no longer than 10 seconds.

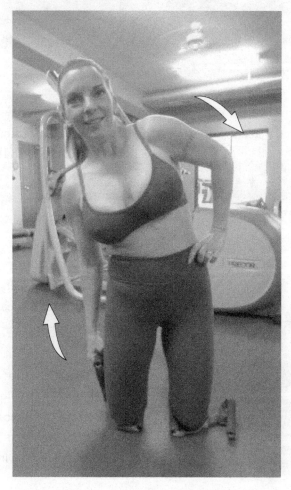

Arms: Biceps and Triceps
Iso-Bow® Biceps and Triceps Cradle Press-Curl
(Left and Right Side)

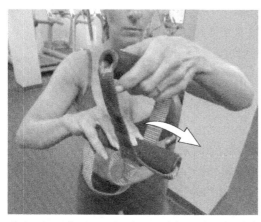

Firstly, you will need to learn how to make an Iso-Bow® cradle.

This is where you effectively half the size of the Iso-Bow® by placing one of the handles inside the webbing loop of the other side of the device. The handle you have just placed inside the loop

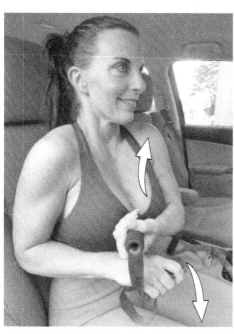

is then cradled by the webbing and can be gripped as normal. Your thumb and fingers can then wrap around both the foam handle and the webbing of the cradle loop to help ensure a firm grip position is created.

To perform the exercises, cradle the Iso-Bow® with

your left hand, gripping the top and with your left hand facing upwards.

Grip the cradled side of the Iso-Bow® with the right hand facing down. Keep both elbows close to your body, and with your left arm across the front of you at waist height.

In this position, press down with the right hand, and at the same time press up with the left. This will engage both the Biceps and Triceps muscles simultaneously.

Breathe naturally and deeply in and out for about 10 full breaths, which will take about 1 second per breath. Aim to perform an exercise breathing count of no less than 7 seconds, and no longer than 10 seconds.

Repeat the same exercise for the other arm by simply reversing the process.

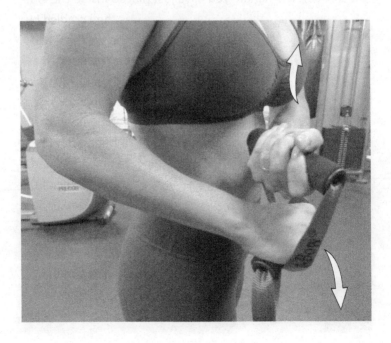

Alternative Biceps and Triceps Dual Exercises Without an Iso-Bow® *(Change Sides & Reverse Grip)*

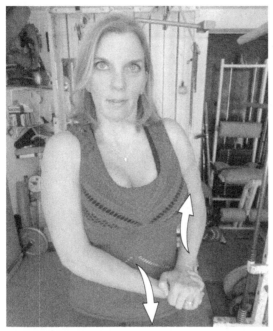

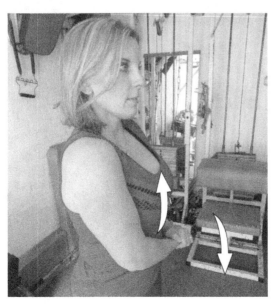

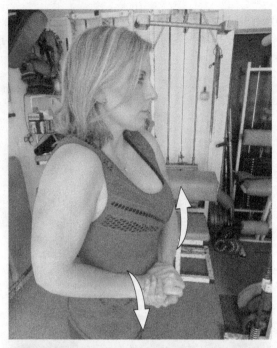
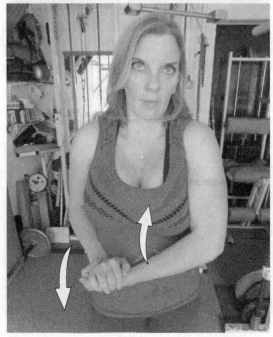

Iso-Bow® Single Arms Biceps Curl – Both Arms

Form a loop on one side of the Iso-Bow® handle as shown, place it around your left foot, and put your left foot on a solid object such as a bench or a chair.

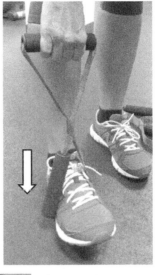

Lean forward and grip the Iso-Bow® handle with your left hand facing up, bracing yourself with your free hand against the bent knee. Try to pull the Iso-Bow® up to engage the biceps muscles, with your foot resisting the exercise.

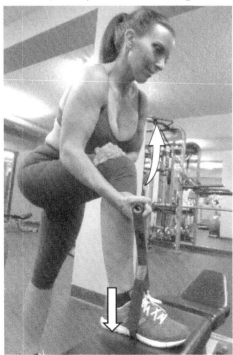

Breathe naturally and deeply in and out for about 10 full breaths, which will take about 1 second per breath. Aim to perform an exercise breathing count of no less than 7 seconds, and no longer than 10 seconds.

Change over hands to perform the same exercise with the other arm.

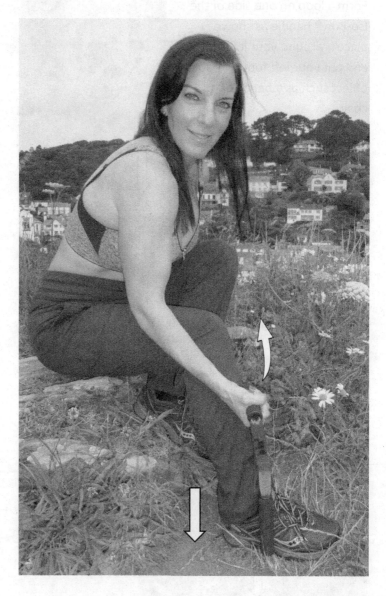

Dual Iso-Bow® Foot Loop Biceps Curl

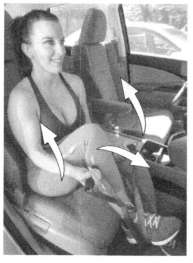

Stand, sit on a chair, or any other solid object. Raise one leg and place the Iso-Bows® around each foot as shown.

In that position, pull up to engage the Biceps, while at the same time pushing the foot down to provide immovable resistance.

Breathe naturally and deeply in and out for about 10 full breaths, which will take about 1 second per breath. Aim to perform an exercise breathing count of no less than 7 seconds, and no longer than 10 seconds.

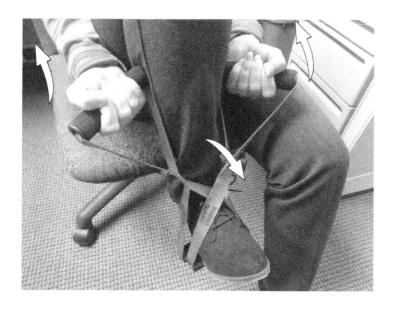

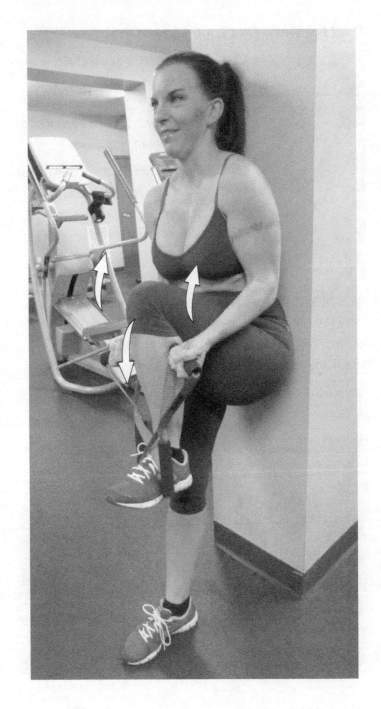

Iso-Bow® Shin-Resisted **Biceps Curl**

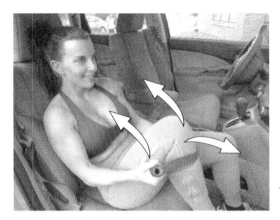

Stand, or sit on a chair, or any other solid object. Raise one leg and place the Iso-Bow® comfortably just below the knee.

Pull up to engage the Biceps muscles of both arms, using the knee and leg to provide immovable resistance.

Breathe naturally and deeply in and out for about 10 full breaths, which will take about 1 second per breath.

Aim to perform an exercise breathing count of no less than 7 seconds, and no longer than 10 seconds.

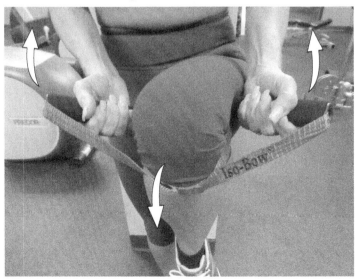

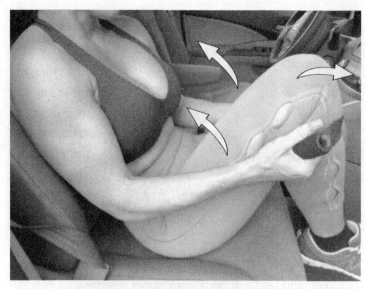
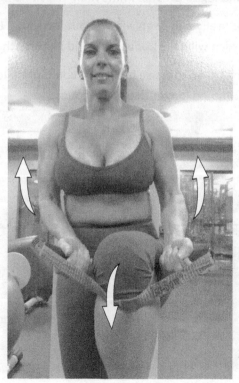

Iso-Bow® Triceps Front Press - Both Arms

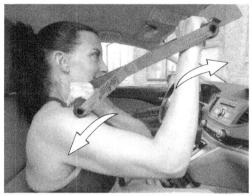

Hold the Iso-Bow® up to your shoulder and grip the handle firmly.

Hold the other handle with your hand facing away from you, keeping your arm and elbow at a 90-degree angle.

Hold the Iso-Bow® up to your shoulder and grip the handle firmly. Hold the other handle with your hand facing away from you, keeping your arm and elbow at a 90-degree angle.

Breathe naturally and deeply in and out for about 10 full breaths, which will take about 1 second per breath.

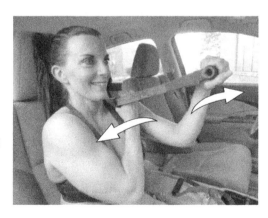

Aim to perform an exercise breathing count of no less than 7 seconds, and no longer than 10 seconds.

Repeat on the other side/arm by reversing the action.

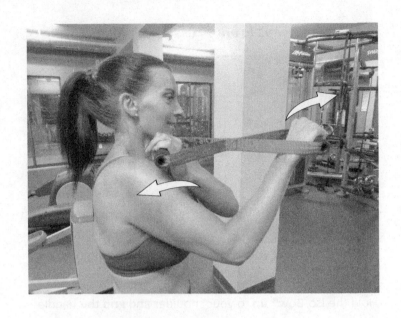

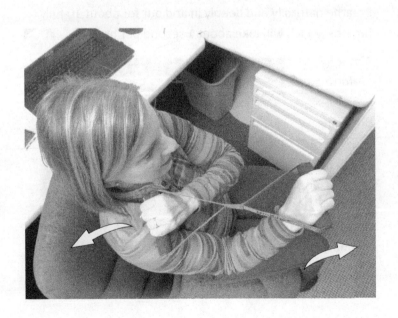

Iso-Bow® Triceps Press Down Over Knee

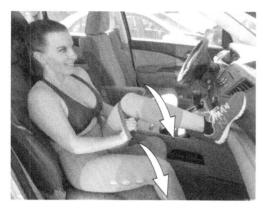

Put one foot on any solid object such as a chair, bench, the dashboard of a car or the seat in front of you. Hold both handles as you place the Iso-Bow® in a comfortable position face downwards over the lower thigh, close to the knee. Bend the arms and lean forward over the knee. Keep your elbows close to your body and push down on each handle to engage the triceps muscles of both arms as you attempt to push your body backwards. You will not be able to move, because your bodyweight and your upper body muscles will provide resistance and prevent you from doing so. Breathe naturally and deeply in and out for about 10 full breaths, which will take about 1 second per breath. Aim to perform an exercise breathing count of no less than 7 seconds, and no longer than 10 seconds.

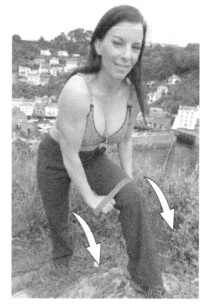

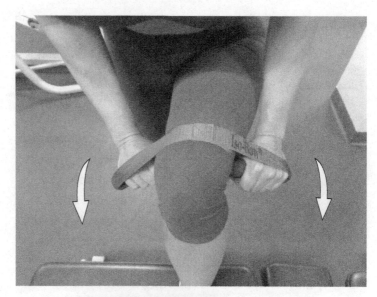
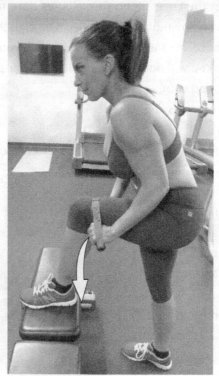

Forearms: Iso-Bow® Wrist Curl and Extension

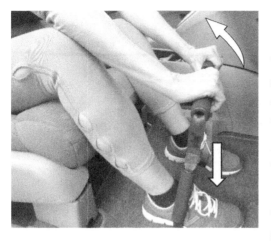

Place an Iso-Bow® around the foot as shown and grip each handle with your palms facing down.

In this position, curl the gripping hand/s upwards to engage the extensor muscles of the upper forearm. Breathe naturally and deeply in and out for about 10 full breaths, which will take about 1 second per breath. Aim to perform an exercise breathing count of no less than 7 seconds, and no longer than 10 seconds.

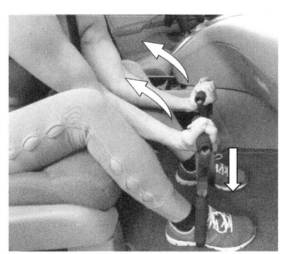

Switch your grip so that your palms are facing up and curl the gripping hand upwards to repeat the exercise for the flexor muscles of your inner forearm.

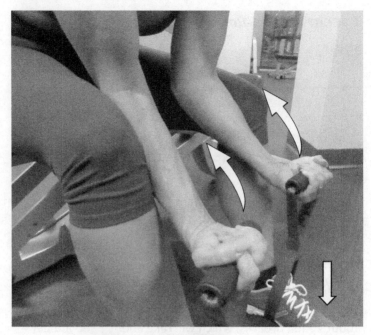
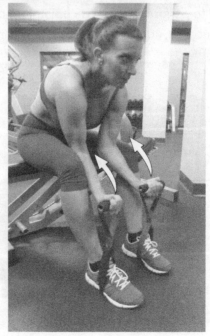

Alternative Exercises Without an Iso-Bow®
(Change sides to exercise both forearms in each direction)

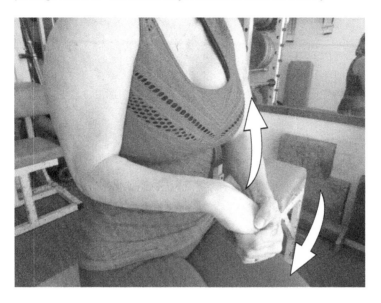

Reverse Hand Position

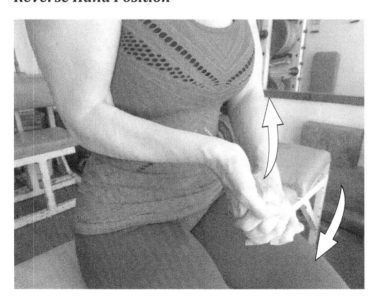

Upper Back
Iso-Bow® Latissimus Overhead Pull Apart

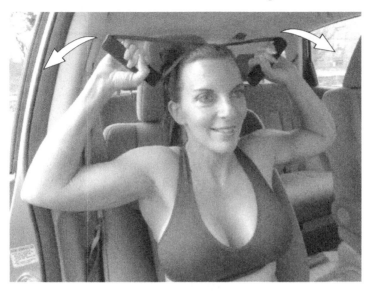

Grip the Iso-Bow® handle, placing the central section comfortably and flat, just above the top of the head.

In this position, try to pull your hands apart, engaging the latissimus muscles of the upper back as you do so.

Breathe naturally and deeply in and out for

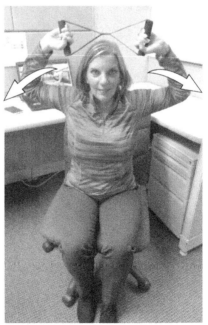

about 10 full breaths, which will take about 1 second per breath.

Aim to perform an exercise breathing count of no less than 7 seconds, and no longer than 10 seconds.

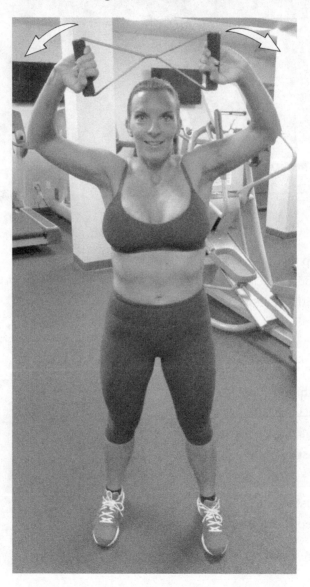

Alternative Exercise Without an Iso-Bow®

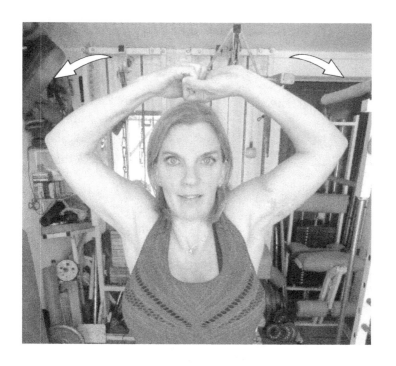

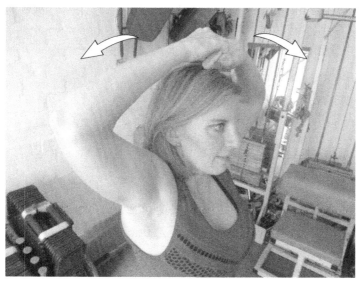

Iso-Bow® Doorway Pull-Ups
ONLY PERFORM IF IT IS SAFE TO DO SO ON A SOLID DOOR.

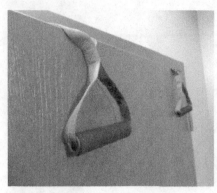

Place the handle of each Iso-Bow® over the top of a solid door as shown, at about shoulder-width apart, close the door and double-check that it is secure.

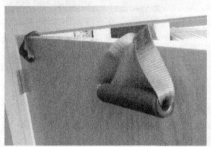

Holding each handle, pull yourself up so that you slide up against the door until your elbows are bent at about a 90-degree angle. Hold this position to engage the upper back muscles as you attempt to pull upwards and forwards as you press against the door which will prevent you from moving.

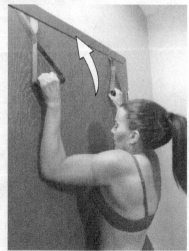

Breathe naturally and deeply in and out for about 10 full breaths, which will take about 1 second per breath. Aim to perform an exercise breathing count of no less than 7 seconds, and no longer than 10 seconds.

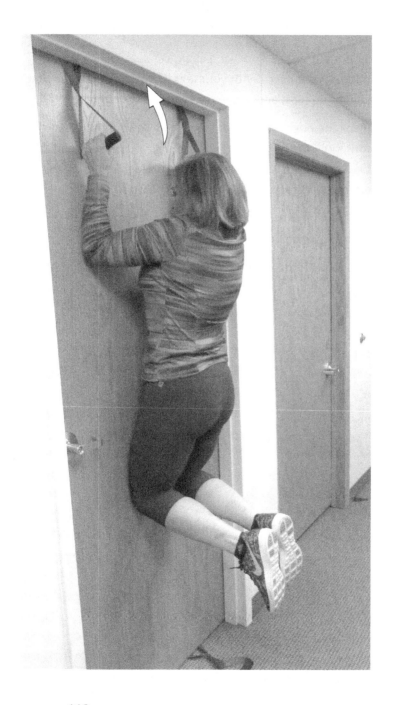

Dual Iso-Bow® Seated Foot-Stirrup Row

Sit upright on the floor, or a chair, car seat, bench, or any other solid object. With your legs in front of you, bend your knees and hips, and always keep your back straight.

Place the one looped end of each Iso-Bow® around each foot, hold the handles firmly, and pull your elbows and arms back to engage your upper back muscles, be sure to keep your elbows close to your body as you do so.

Breathe naturally and deeply in and out for about 10 full breaths, which will take about 1 second per breath.

Aim to perform an exercise breathing count of no less than 7 seconds, and no longer than 10 seconds.

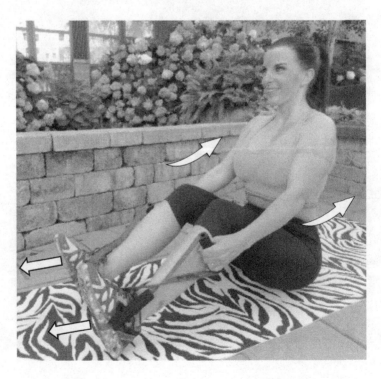

Dual Iso-Bow® Seated Foot Stirrup Row

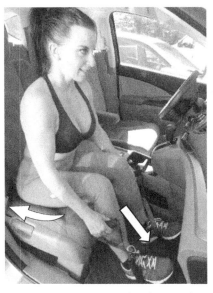

Sit on a chair, or any other solid object, with your feet on the floor in front of you, and bend your knees and hips, while keeping your back straight.

Place one of the looped ends of each Iso-Bow® around each foot, hold the handles firmly, and pull your elbows and arms back to engage your upper back muscles, be sure to keep your elbows close to your body as you do so.

Breathe naturally and deeply in and out for about 10 full

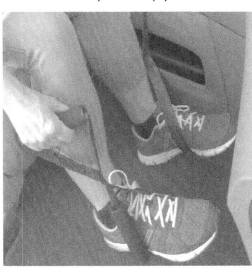

breaths, which will take about 1 second per breath. Aim to perform an exercise breathing count of no less than 7 seconds, and no longer than 10.

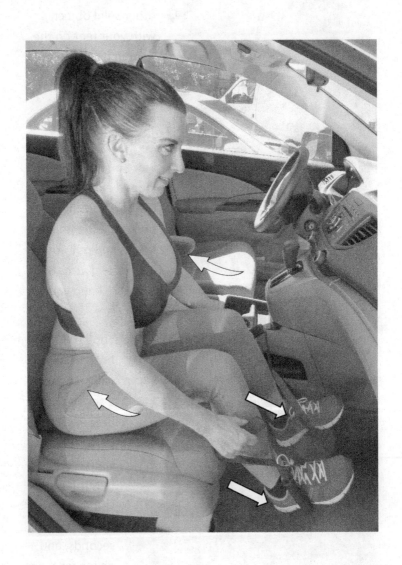

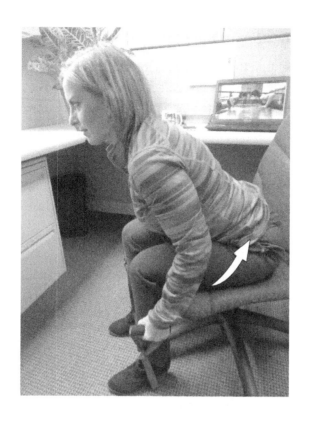
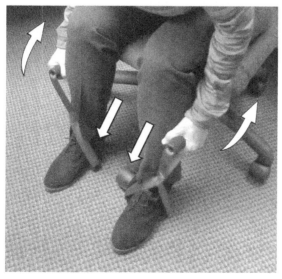

Iso-Bow® Upper Back Seated Knee Brace Row

Sit upright on the floor, bench, or seat. If necessary, with your feet under a secure object that will not tip over. Bend forward only from the hips and keep your back straight.

Wrap the Iso-Bow® comfortably around both knees and lean your upper body backwards slightly.

At the same time, pull back with each handle to engage your upper back muscles, keeping your elbows close to your body as you do so.

This will naturally begin to bring your upper body into a more upright position where you can begin the isometric exercise.

Breathe naturally and deeply in and out for about 10 full breaths, which will take about 1 second per breath.

Aim to perform an exercise breathing count of no less than 7 seconds, and no longer than 10 seconds.

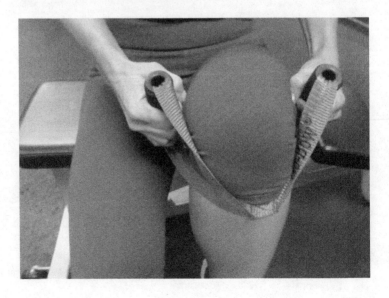

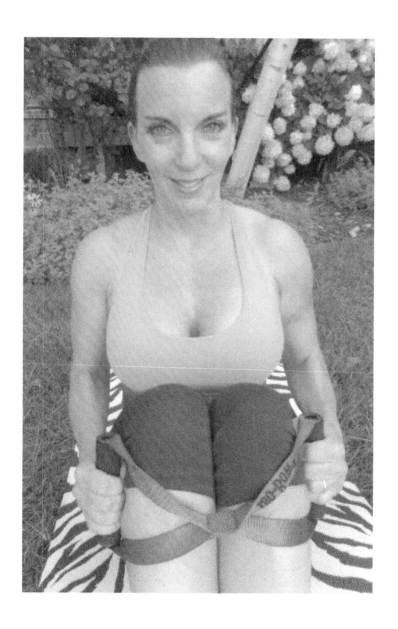

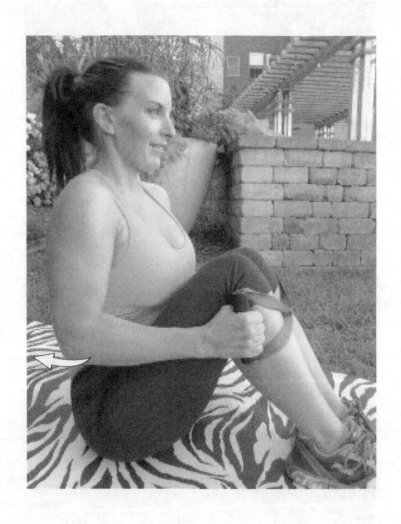

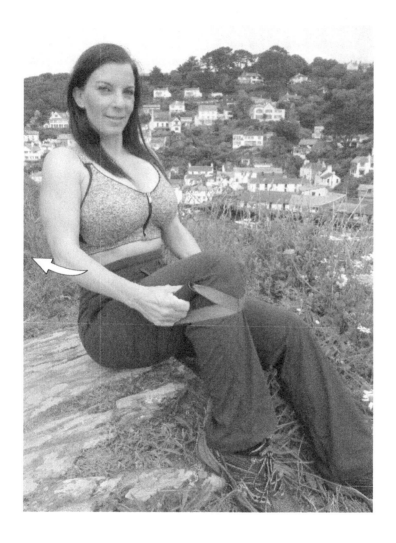

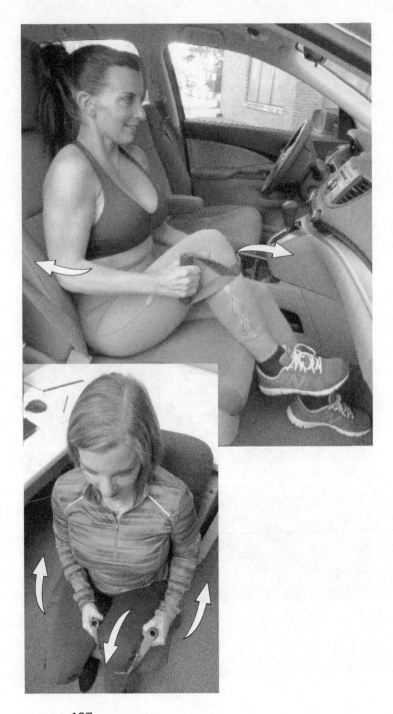

Alternative Exercise Without an Iso-Bow®

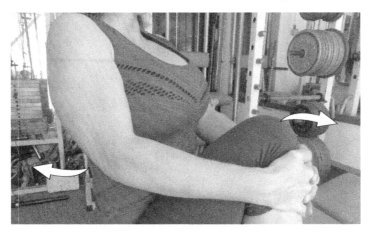

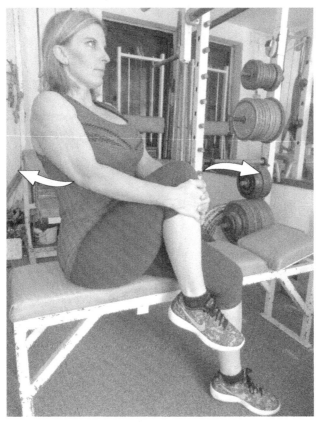

Iso-Bow® Back Power Cradle-Pull Apart Wide

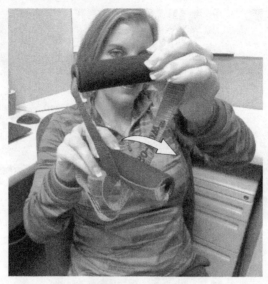

Firstly, cradle the Iso-Bow® to effectively half its size.

Then, hold the Iso-Bow® in front of you, with your arms bent, and approximately parallel to the floor. In this position, attempt to pull the Iso-Bow® apart to engage the central upper back muscles.

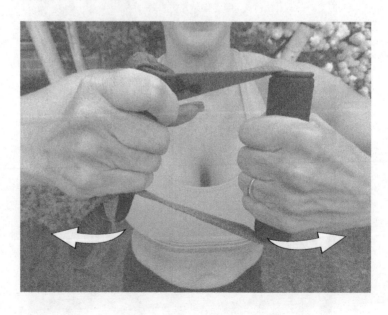

Breathe naturally and deeply in and out for about 10 full breaths, which will take about 1 second per breath. Aim to perform an exercise breathing count of no less than 7 seconds, and no longer than 10 seconds.

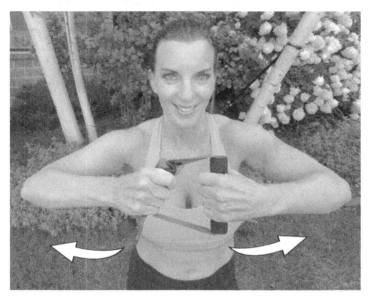

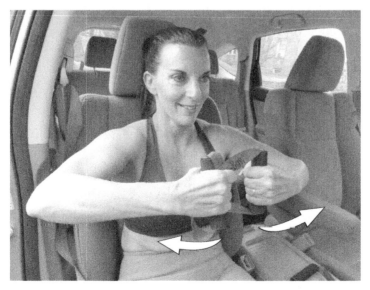

Iso-Bow® Back Power Pull-Apart Wide

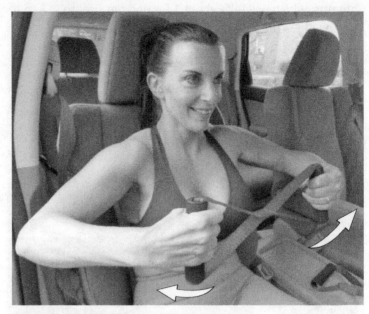

Hold the Iso-Bow® in front of you, with your arms bent, and approximately parallel to the floor.

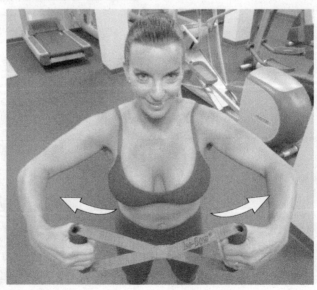

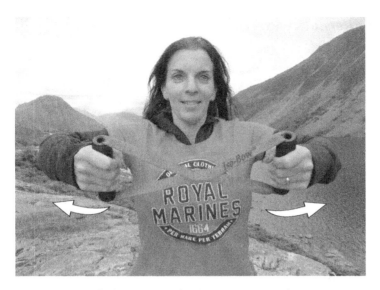

Attempt to pull the Iso-Bow® apart to engage the upper back muscles. Breathe naturally and deeply in and out for about 10 full breaths, which will take about 1 second per breath. Aim to perform an exercise breathing count of no less than 7 seconds, and no longer than 10 seconds.

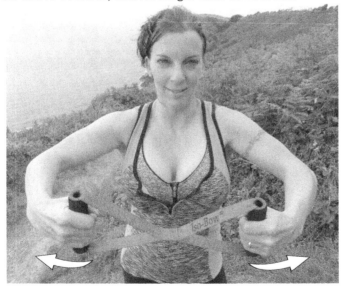

Alternative Exercise Without an Iso-Bow®

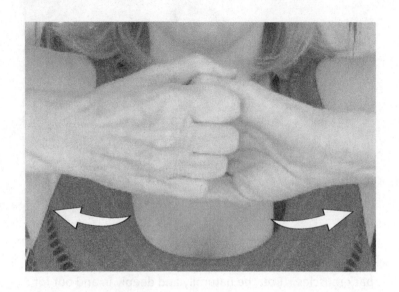

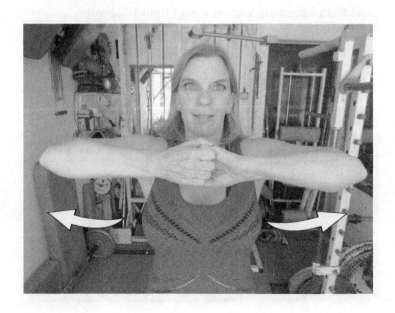

Iso-Bow® Archer Row – Right and Left Side

With one arm in front of you roughly parallel to the floor, push one end of the Iso-Bow® forward. At the same time, pull the other handle backwards to 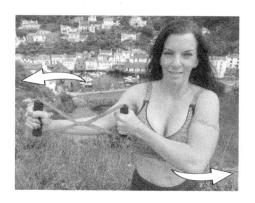 engage the upper back muscles on that side of the body.

Breathe naturally and deeply in and out for about 10 full breaths, which will take about 1 second per breath. Aim to perform an exercise breathing count of no less than 7 seconds, and no longer than 10 seconds.

Reverse the handgrip positions to exercise the upper back muscles on the other side of your torso.

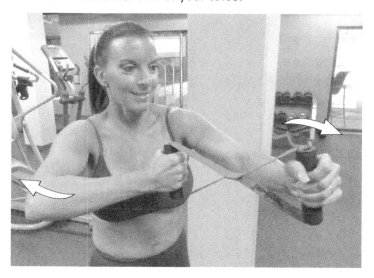

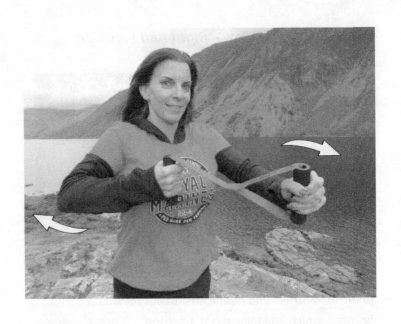

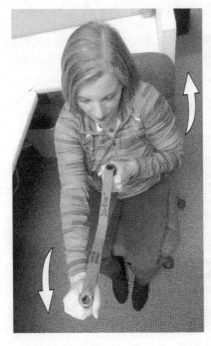

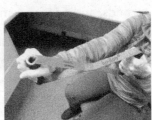

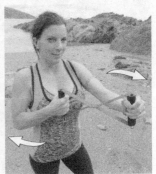

135

Lower Back: Dual Iso-Bow® Bent-Leg Deadlift

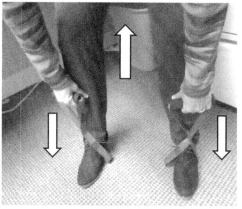

Place the loop handle of each Iso-Bow® around each foot as shown. Hold both handles firmly, while maintaining a perfect bent-knee, semi-squat position. With your back straight, attempt to slowly stand up straight. As you do so, engage the muscles of the glutes, hamstrings, lower back, thighs, and other core muscles. At the same time, the Iso-Bows®, secured by your feet, prevent any further movement from taking place.

Breathe naturally and deeply in and out for about 10 full breaths, which will take about 1 second per breath.

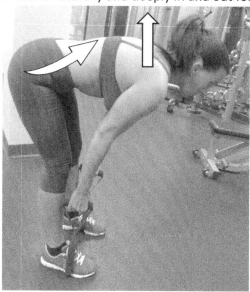

Aim to perform an exercise breathing count of no less than 7 seconds, and no longer than 10 seconds.

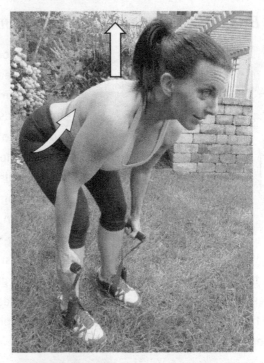

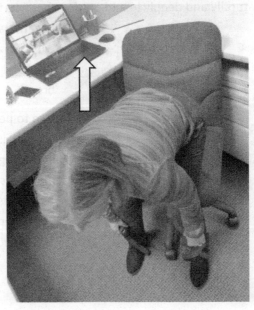

Iso-Bow® Intermediate Lower Back Extension

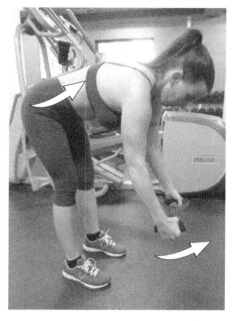

Stand with your feet shoulder-width apart, and with your knees slightly bent. Bend forwards only from the hips as low as you are comfortably able to and hold both handles of an Iso-Bow® downwards towards the floor.

To increase the force and intensity on the lower back muscles, in the same position extend your arms forward, and hold the Iso-Bow® straight out in front of you as far as you are comfortable. Breathe naturally and deeply in and out for about 10 full breaths, which will take about 1 second per breath. Aim to perform an exercise breathing count of no less than 7 seconds, and no longer than 10 seconds.

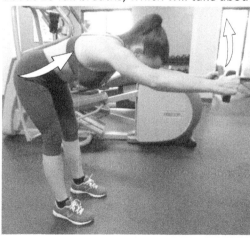

A more advanced lower back exercise can be performed by lying on the floor, face down. Simultaneously raise both arms in the extended position as shown below, while raising both feet/legs as well.

All exercises in the intermediate lower back section can be performed with or without an Iso-Bow®.

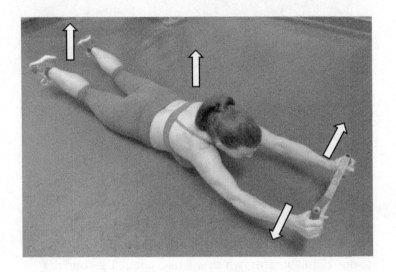

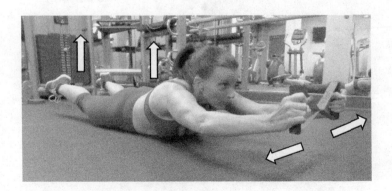

Chest: Iso-Bow® Cradle Cross Press

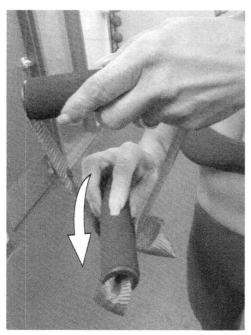

Cradle the Iso-Bow® to make a shorter handgrip.

Cross it in front of you at chest level, with your arms roughly parallel to the floor, and push in opposing directions sideways to engage your chest muscles.

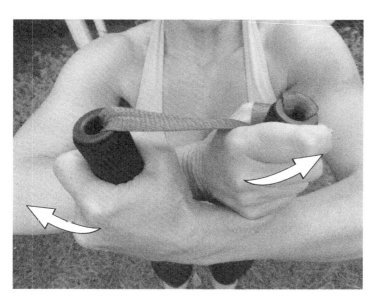

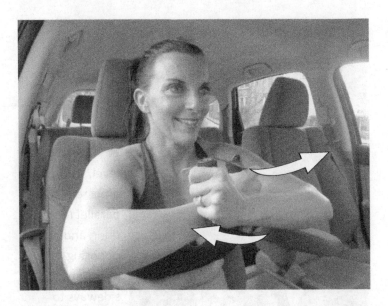

Breathe naturally and deeply in and out for about 10 full breaths, which will take about 1 second per breath.

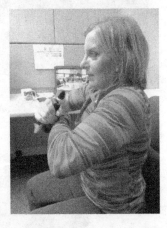

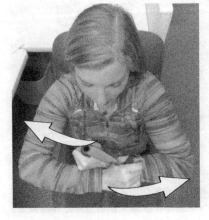

Aim to perform an exercise breathing count of no less than 7 seconds, and no longer than 10 seconds.

Iso-Bow® Chest Cross Press Wide

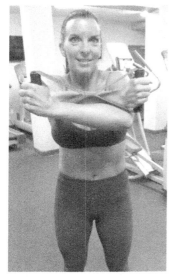

Cross the Iso-Bow® in front of you at chest level, with your arms roughly parallel to the floor. Push in opposing directions sideways, to engage your chest muscles. Breathe naturally and deeply in and out for about 10 full breaths, which will take about 1 second per breath. Aim to perform an exercise breathing count of no less than 7 seconds, and no longer than 10 seconds.

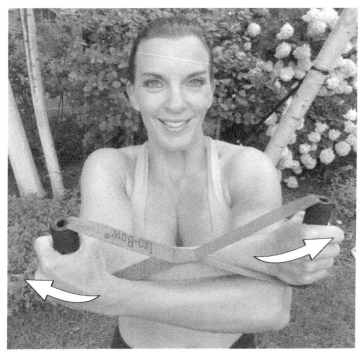

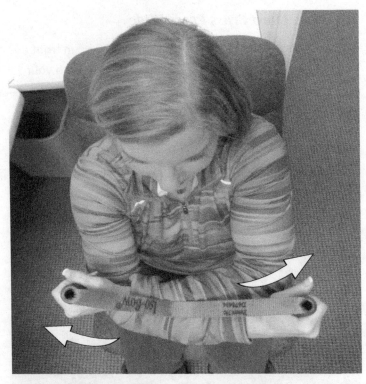
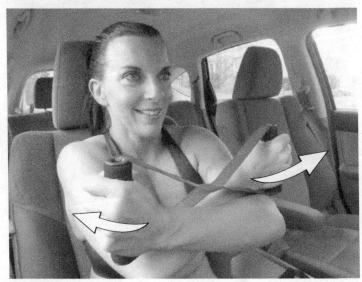

Alternative Chest Exercise Without an Iso-Bow®

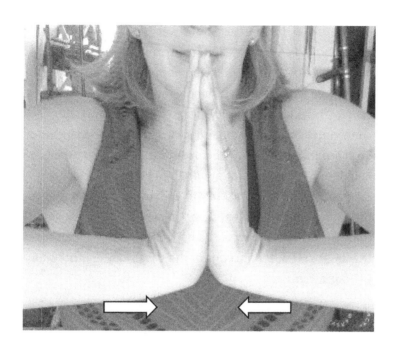

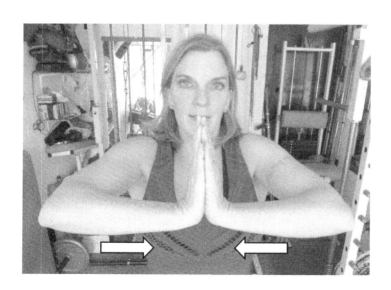

Iso-Bow® Chest Press Inner and Outer Push

With one arm in front of you roughly parallel to the floor, push one end of the Iso-Bow® forward. As you do so, keep your elbow slightly bent, and focus your push slightly inwards, across to the centre point of the chest. At the same time, push the other handle inwards, and across your chest. This exercise should engage the inner and outer chest muscles at the same time. Always keep the elbows of both arms slightly during the exercise. Breathe naturally and deeply in and out for about 10 full breaths, which will take about 1 second per breath. Aim to perform an exercise breathing count of no less than 7 seconds, and no longer than 10 seconds. Reverse the handgrip positions to exercise the inner and outer portions of the chest on the other side of your torso.

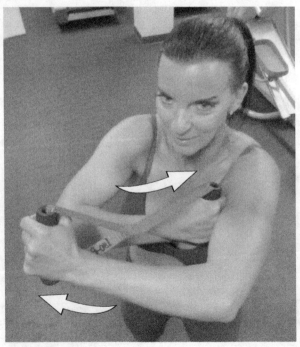

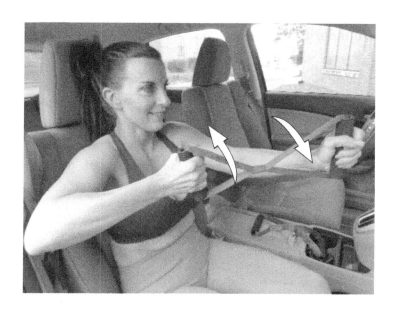

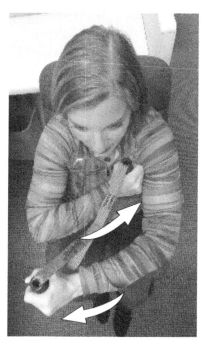
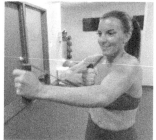
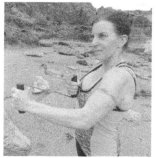

Dual Iso-Bow® Power Push

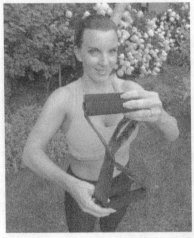

Wrap two Iso-Bows® together as shown. Hold the 4 combined handles, in a comfortable and firm position with the handles sitting low in the palms of each hand, near the wrists.

Press the combined Iso-Bows® together to engage your chest muscles, with your arms roughly parallel to the floor as you attempt to compress the immovable handles.

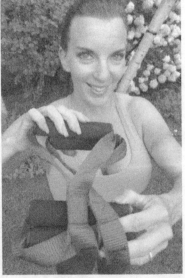

Breathe naturally and deeply in and out for about 10 full breaths, which will take about 1 second per breath.

Aim to perform an exercise breathing count

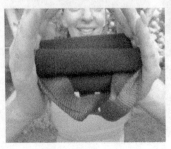

of no less than 7 seconds, and no longer than 10 seconds.

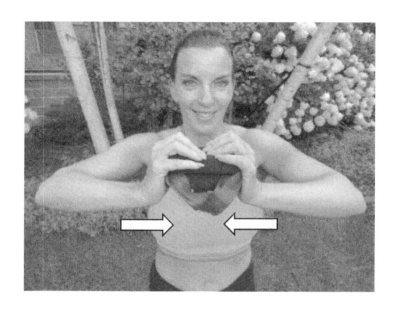

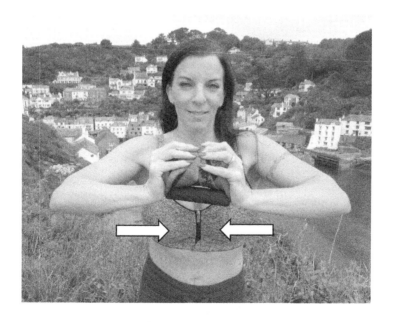

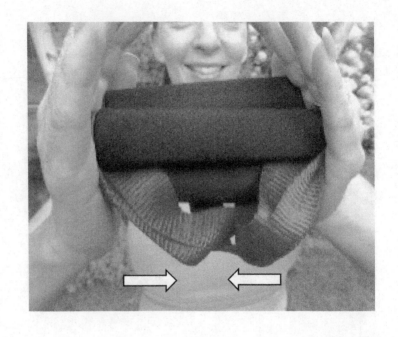

Shoulders:
Iso-Bow® Overhead Press – Left and Right Arm

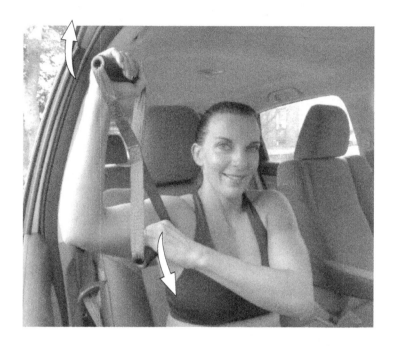

Hold one end of the Iso-Bow® in your upper hand, ensuring that your arm always stays at an angle of approximately 90 degrees.

Push upwards, as if to perform a shoulder press, and resist the movement by pulling back and downwards with the opposing hand and arm.

Breathe naturally and deeply in and out for about 10 full breaths, which will take about 1 second per breath.

Aim to perform an exercise breathing count of no less than 7 seconds, and no longer than 10 seconds. Then repeat the exercise on the other side for the other shoulder.

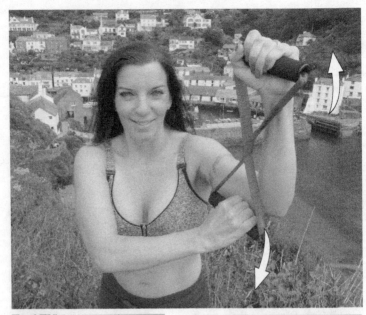
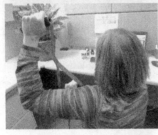
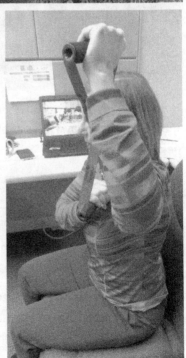
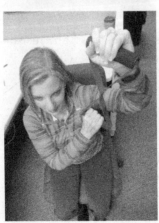

Iso-Bow® Front Raise - Left and Right Arm

Hold each handle of the Iso-Bow® firmly in front of you as shown. Keep your leading elbow slightly bent and use the front shoulder muscles to resist the downward pull of the lower hand and arm.

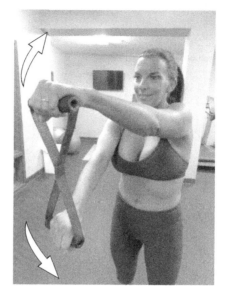

Breathe naturally and deeply in and out for about 10 full breaths, which will take about 1 second per breath. Aim to perform an exercise breathing count of no less than 7 seconds, and no longer than 10 seconds. Repeat the exercise on the other side by reversing the hand and arm positions.

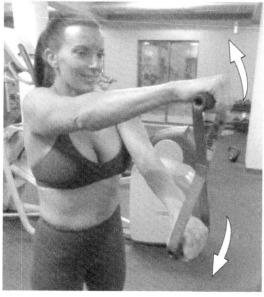

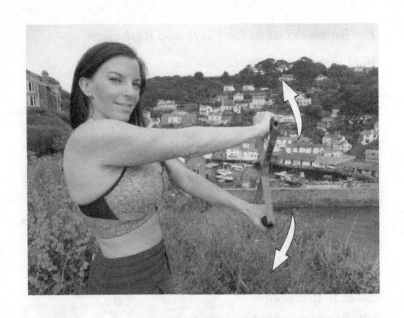
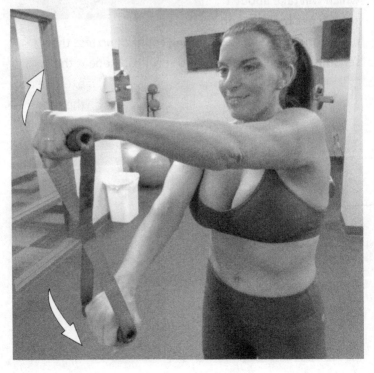

Iso-Bow® Side Lateral Raise – Both Sides

Hold the Iso-Bow® slightly to one side with both hands, roughly halfway between lap and shoulder level, keeping your elbows very slightly bent.

The elbow of the raised arm should be kept high, to properly engage only the side deltoids. Attempt to pull the Iso-Bow® down with your lower arm, while resisting

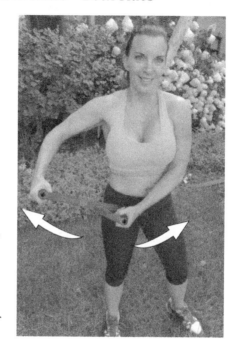

and engaging the side shoulder muscles, or deltoids, of the higher arm as you do so.

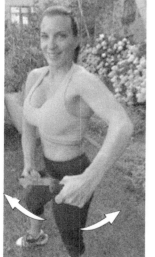

Breathe naturally and deeply in and out for about 10 full breaths, which will take about 1 second per breath.

Aim to perform an exercise breathing count of no less than 7 seconds, and no longer than 10 seconds. Then repeat the exercise on the other side by reversing the hand and arm positions.

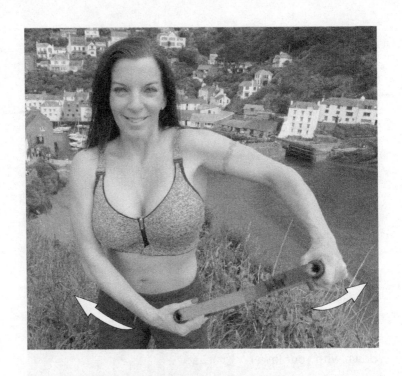

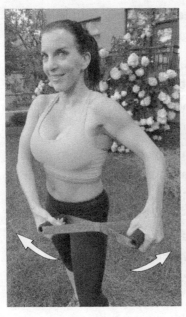 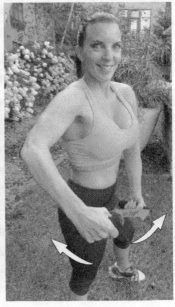

Iso-Bow® Mid Hold Lateral Raise Pull-Apart

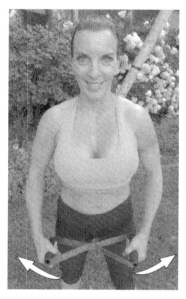

Hold the Iso-Bow® in both hands, at lap level in front of you, and with your elbows very slightly bent. In this position, attempt to pull it apart by raising both arms sideways, and engaging the side shoulder muscles, or deltoids, as you do so. Breathe naturally and deeply in and out for about 10 full breaths, which will take about 1 second per breath.

Aim to perform an exercise breathing count of no less than 7 seconds, and no longer than 10 seconds.

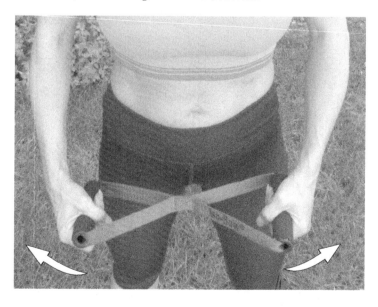

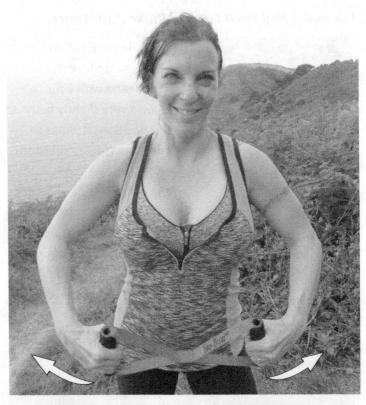
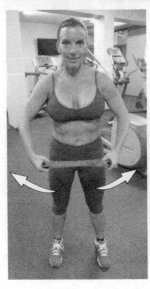
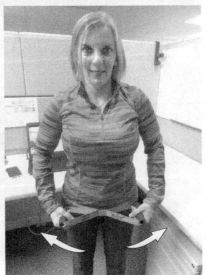

Alternative Exercises Without an Iso-Bow®
(To Exercise Both Shoulders, Change Leading Hand to Alternate Side)

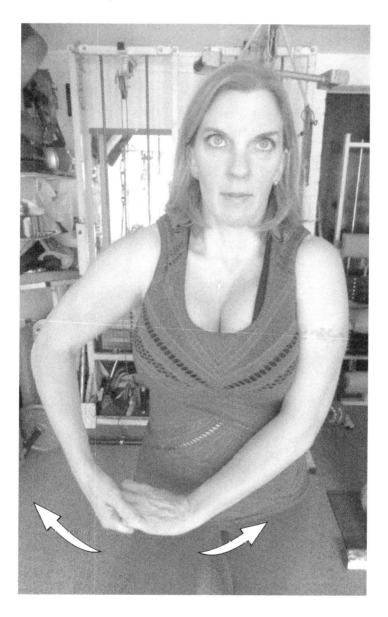

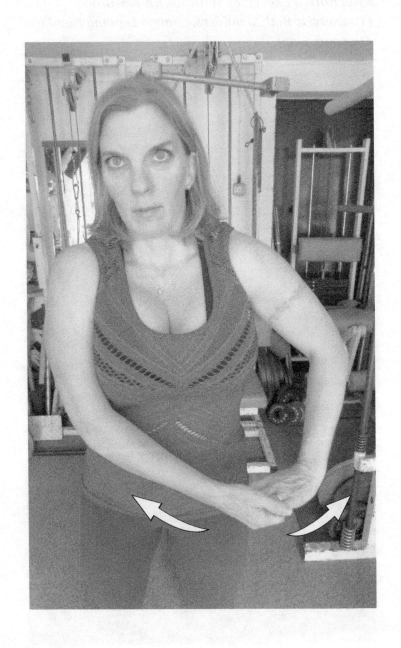

Legs: Upper Thighs
Iso-Bow® Leg Extension – Left and Right Leg

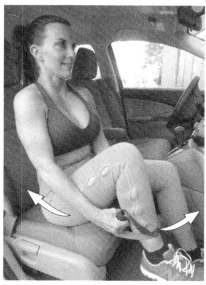

Sit on a chair, or any other solid object, raise one knee and place the Iso-Bow® comfortably around the lower part of your leg, close to your foot.

Hold both handles firmly, keep your back straight, bend only from the hips, and lean back slightly as you try to extend your foot forward while keeping your toes pointing upwards.

Breathe naturally and deeply in and out for about 10 full breaths, which will take about 1 second per breath.

Aim to perform an exercise breathing count of no less than

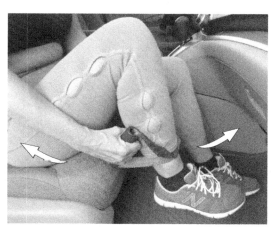

7 seconds, and no longer than 10 seconds. Switch legs and repeat the exercise with the other leg.

As an alternative to using your lower shin to resist the Iso-Bow®, you can equally easily loop one foot, through one handle of each Iso-Bow® as shown. Keeping your toes pulled upwards, engage the thigh muscles by applying pressure to extend the foot forwards, and slightly upwards.

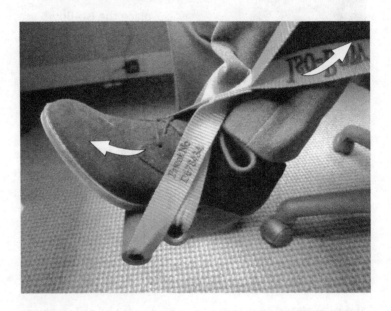

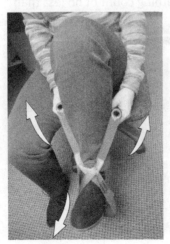

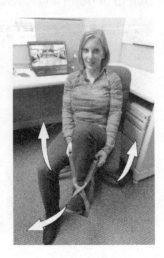

Alternative Exercise Without an Iso-Bow®

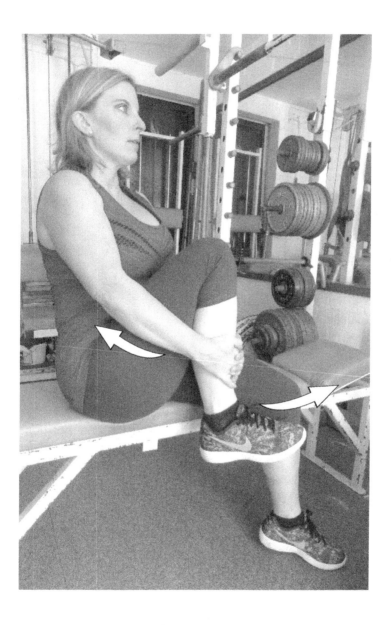

Dual Iso-Bow® Stirrup Squat

Place one looped handle side of each Iso-Bow® around each foot as shown.

Bend your torso forward and only at the hips, always keeping your back straight and upright.

Grip each Iso-Bow® handle firmly and attempt to stand upright from your chair by engaging your upper thigh and glute muscles. You can always perform this exercise without a chair, by starting in the standing position.

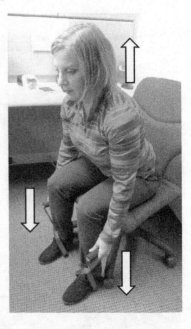

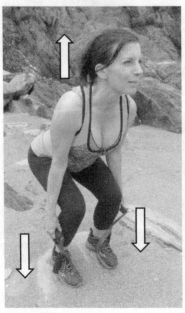

Naturally, you will not be able to move but continue your attempt to stand up, while maintaining the perfect mid-squat position as you do so. Breathe naturally and deeply in and out for about 10 full breaths, which will take about 1 second per breath. Aim to perform an exercise breathing count of no less than 7 seconds, and no longer than 10 seconds.

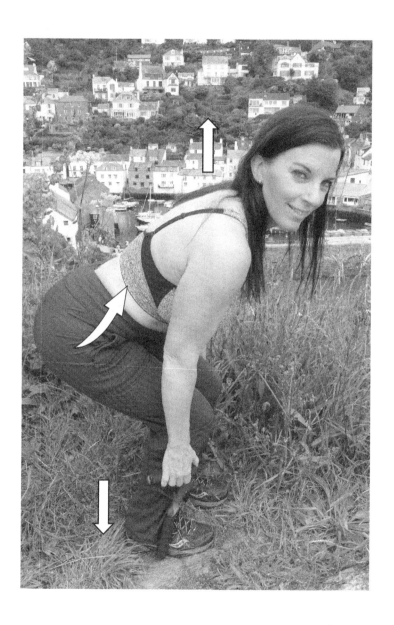

Alternative Exercise Without an Iso-Bow®

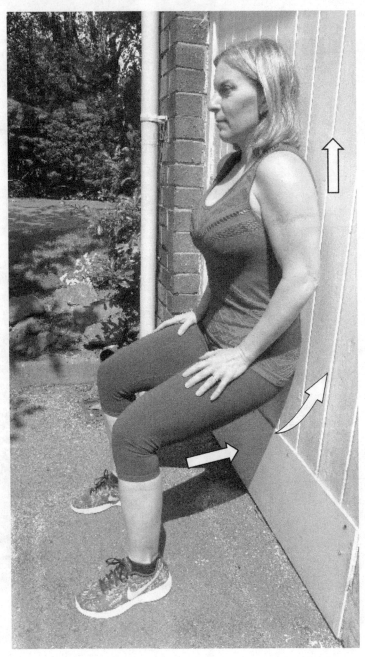

Iso-Bow® Forward Split Squat - Left and Right Leg

Place the looped ends of two Iso-Bows® around the foot as shown to make a double stirrup. Bend one knee forward to about a 90-degree angle and move the other leg backward. Keep your trailing knee close to the floor, to create a split squat position. Hold both Iso-Bow® handles firmly, and keeping your body upright, and your back 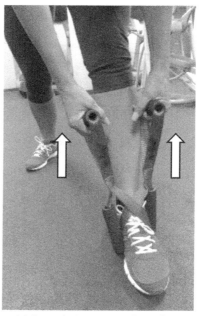 straight, use and engage the thigh and glute muscles of your leading leg as you attempt to straighten it and push 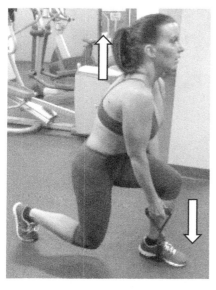 upwards. Breathe naturally and deeply in and out for about 10 full breaths, which will take about 1 second per breath. Aim to perform an exercise breathing count of no less than 7 seconds, and no longer than 10 seconds. Repeat the exercise with the other leg.

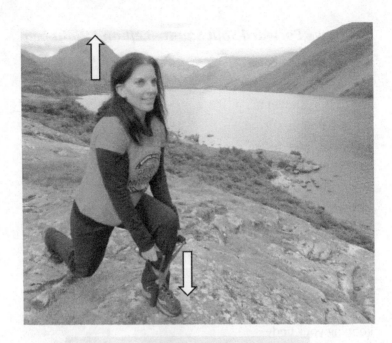
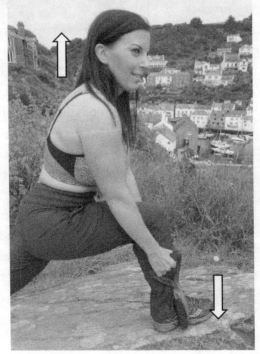

Iso-Bow® Hamstring Seated Curl – Both Legs

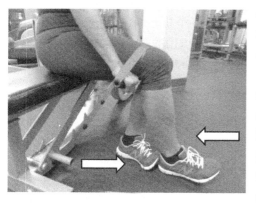

Sit on a chair, car seat or bench, and push the Iso-Bow® comfortably down over one leg to help prevent it from rising during the exercise.

Place one foot directly in front of the other, so the heel of the leading foot is touching the toes of your rear foot and

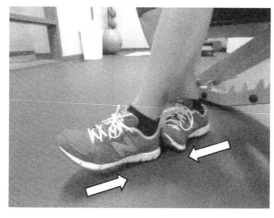

turn up the toes to create a firmer connection.

Try to draw back the leading foot by engaging the hamstring muscles of the rear upper thigh.

Breathe naturally and deeply in and out for about 10 full breaths, which will take about 1 second per breath.

Aim to perform an exercise breathing count of no less than 7 seconds, and no longer than 10 seconds. Repeat the exercise for the other leg, by swapping the leg and foot positions.

The hamstring curl exercise can also be performed against a wall or a door. Standing upright, lean your whole body against the door, then position the heel of one foot against the object to engage the hamstrings as you attempt to curl the foot back against the immovable object.

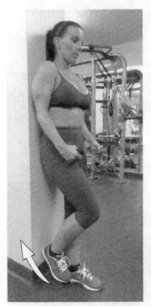
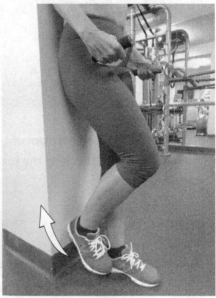
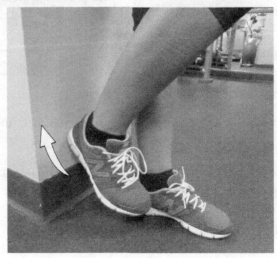

Alternative Exercise Without an Iso-Bow®

By pushing forward by engaging the rear leg/foot, and pushing back with the leading leg/foot, it becomes a dual front upper thigh and rear upper thigh exercise.

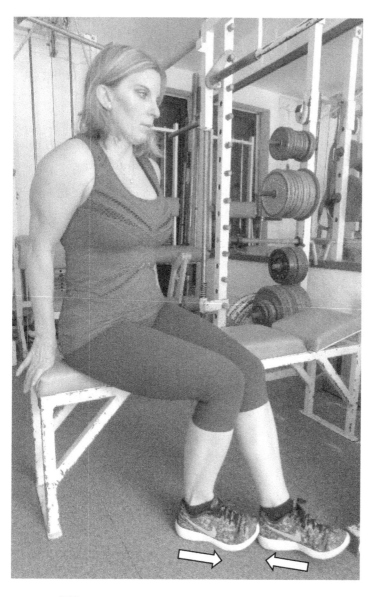

Iso-Bow® Foot Loop **Abductor**

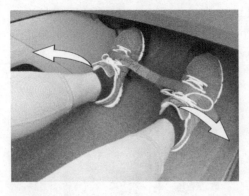

Place each of the Iso-Bow® handles around your feet as shown, and lean back on a chair, any solid object, or flat on the floor.

Lift your legs slightly off the floor, and pull your feet apart, sideways to engage the outer thigh, hip, and glute muscles.

Breathe naturally and deeply in and out for about 10 full breaths, which will take about 1 second per breath.

Aim to perform an exercise breathing count of no less than 7 seconds, and no longer than 10 seconds.

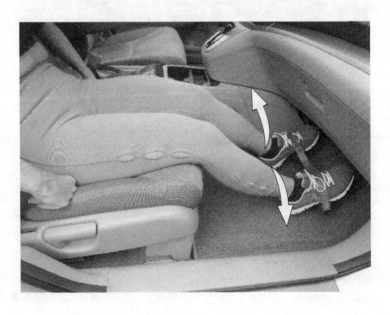

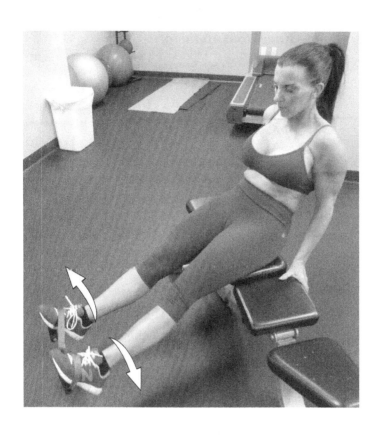

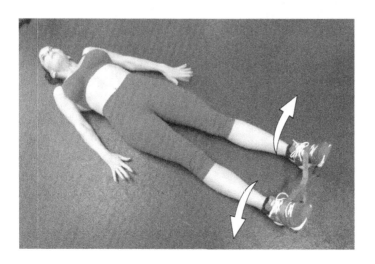

Iso-Bow® Knee Hold Abductor

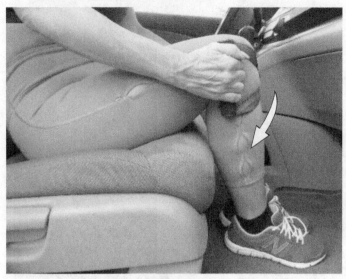

Sit on a chair, car seat, bench, or any other solid object and place the Iso-Bow® around the knees as shown. Hold the handles as you attempt to pull the knees apart to engage the outer thigh muscles and the glutes. Breathe naturally

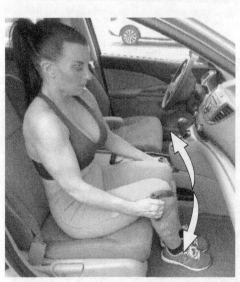

and deeply in and out for about 10 full breaths, which will take about 1 second per breath. Aim to perform an exercise breathing count of no less than 7 seconds, and no longer than 10 seconds.

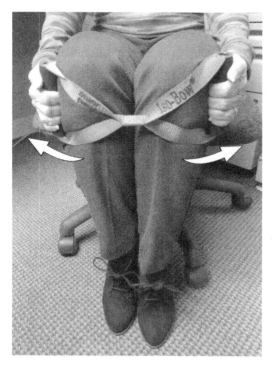

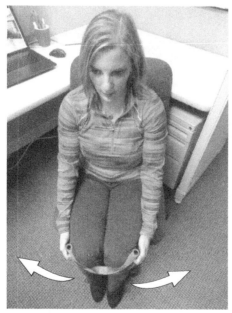

Iso-Bow® Knee-Press Adductor

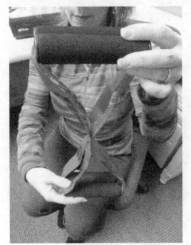

Sit on a chair or any other solid object.

Wrap two Iso-Bows® together to make a four-handle pair, then place them between the knees.

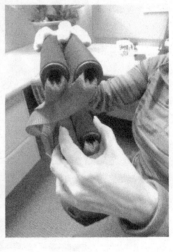

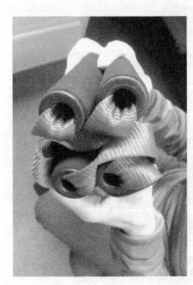

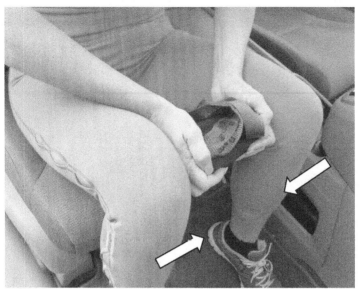

Squeeze the knees together to engage the two Iso-Bows® with inner thigh muscles.

Breathe naturally and deeply in and out for about 10 full breaths, which will take about 1 second per breath.

Aim to perform an exercise breathing count of no less than 7 seconds, and no longer than 10 seconds.

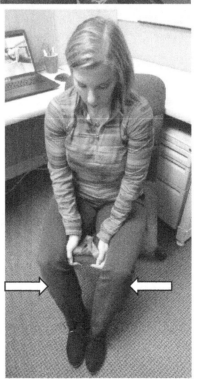

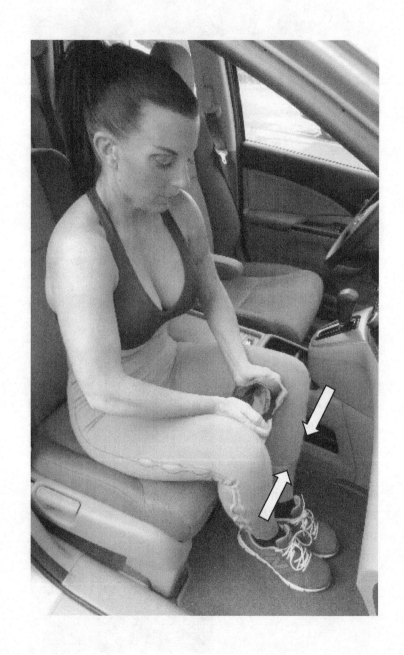

Legs: Calf's

Calf Single Leg Wall Push – Left and Right Leg

Place your hands against a wall, a car, a door frame, or any other solid object which is immovable by human muscle power alone. With one leg back in a firm position and with the ball of your foot on the floor, raise the heel slightly as you engage your calf muscles, pushing against the immovable object.

Breathe naturally and deeply in and out for about 10 full breaths, which will take about 1 second per breath.

Aim to perform an exercise breathing count of no less than 7 seconds, and no longer than 10 seconds.

Switch legs and repeat the exercise with the other leg.

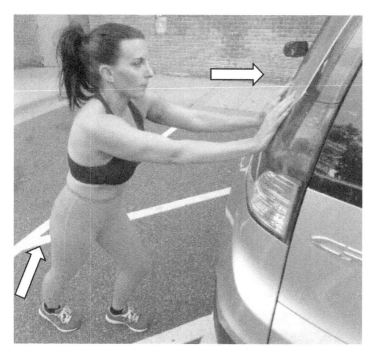

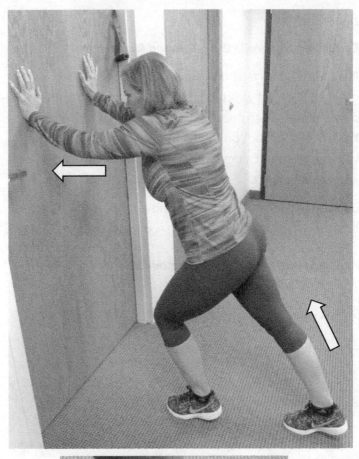
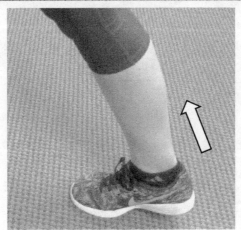

Chapter 8: Conclusion

Your health, strength, fitness, and body shape should not be restricted and disrupted by simply travelling away from home for either business or pleasure. Not being able to exercise in a gym should not be a "forced" limitation that is imposed upon you just because you want to exercise and stay in great shape. That is old-fashioned and restrictive thinking.

Even though many hotels boast that they have a gym/fitness suite, all too often it is a "token gesture" of what most of us would want. Some hotels have even taken something which was once a small storeroom, or large cupboard, and then retrofitted it with the equivalent of a domestic cross trainer, a pair of elastic exercise straps, and a single pair of 5 lb dumbbells. Laughably, doing this, allows them to advertise that they have a "fitness facility." Seriously? This is insulting to common sense, and desperate hotels that do this sort of thing are an embarrassment because the rooms and the equipment they provide are usually scarcely able to accommodate a "Hobbit."

You deserve better. Especially if you take your fitness, strength training, bodybuilding, and body shaping seriously. Today, it is easier than ever to be able to perform an effective improvised workout routine in a hotel room. The chances are that if you do this, then it will almost certainly yield better results than the "broom cupboard" token gesture style of gym.

What we offer with the "Fitness on the Move™" concept, is the opportunity to benefit from a high-level, high-intensity, gym-standard workout session which can easily be performed in a near "Zero Footprint Workout™" environment. The ISOfitness™ system, in conjunction with a pair of incredible Iso-Bow® devices, can deliver high-intensity isometric exercise sessions, advanced TRISOmetric™ exercise sessions, revolutionary Iso-Motion®, and advanced traditional callisthenic exercise sessions. The determining factor about what level, and what intensity of workout you ultimately perform, is "you." "You" make every choice in life deliberately. "You" choose how much, how often, and how intensely you exercise, and therefore, how committed you are to becoming stronger, more muscular, and getting into great shape. The simple "tools" we offer, allow you to do all the above.

Are they the answer to everything, to everyone's requirements and preferences? No, of course, they are not. Nothing ever will be. However, they do deliver far more than most people can imagine. It is unfortunate that many people, and especially many bodybuilders, are some of the most closed-minded people around. They simply do not "want" to believe that you can get a high-intensity workout session unless you lift weights in a gym. They simply cannot comprehend that their muscles being exercised do not actually "know" if the resistance is provided by a dumbbell, barbell, bodyweight, or an Iso-Bow™! Muscles simply respond to exercise, resistance, applied force, and overall intensity, irrespective of the source.

We would like to sincerely thank all open-minded people who have read our book/s and who hopefully use the isometric exercise system! Here's to your continued success and to maintaining your "Fitness on the Move™!"

What is TWiEA™?

For more information and member's online video resources for TWiEA members, visit www.TWiEA.com. TWiEA™ is the acronym for The World Isometric Exercise Association which is the governing body for all types of isometric exercise. Its mission is to help set and maintain standards of excellence in teaching and promoting all types of isometric exercise. TWiEA™ seeks to ensure that scientifically proven isometric exercise techniques are taught as part of an integrated overall approach to the total-body exercise solutions provided by fitness professionals. This creates a much higher probability that busy clients facing real-life time crunches can maintain an effective exercise program. Isometric exercise is every bit as effective at building muscle and strength as other traditional forms of resistance training. It is also a time-saving and money-saving exercise solution that almost anyone can perform without any special equipment.

www.MajorVision.com – www.TWiEA.com

Other books by Brian Sterling-Vete and Helen Renée Wuorio

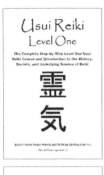

Usui Reiki Level One
A comprehensive introduction to Reiki, its history, and the science. This course is written in an easy-to-follow step-by-step way, so you know exactly what to do and when to do it. This and other books in the series also serve as course manuals for our Reiki students.

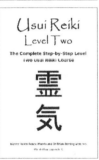

Usui Reiki Level Two
The Reiki Level Two course is the next step in your Reiki journey teaching the Power Symbols and how to use them. It is laid out in an easy-to-understand step-by-step way so you will know exactly what to do and when to do it.

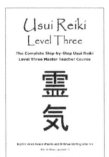

Usui Reiki Level Three
The Level Three Master Teacher course is the final step after Level Two. It is laid out logically in an easy-to-understand step-by-step way so you will know exactly what to do and when to do it.

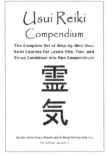

Usui Reiki Compendium – Levels 1 & 2
The Reiki Compendium is a complete and unabridged, book of our Usui Reiki Level One and Two courses. It's ideal for those wishing to progress right through both levels. This and other books in the series also serve as course manuals for our online or in-person Reiki Students.

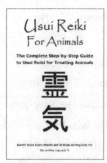

Usui Reiki for Treating Animals

The Usui Reiki for Animals book is ideal for practitioners at any level who want to learn techniques for treating animals of all kinds safely and effectively. It also covers the differences in animal chakras and energy centres as well as others that are unique to certain animals.

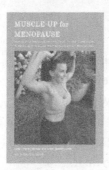

Muscle-up For Menopause

Approved by TWiEA – The World Isometric Exercise Association. Menopause cannot be avoided so take control of every element possible. Brief yet intense exercise sessions that place the minimum demand on your ability to recover combined with a high-protein plant-based diet can make all the difference between making life easier or harder during menopause. This course can be performed with or without equipment.

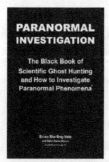

Paranormal Investigation - The Black Book of Scientific Ghost Hunting and How to Investigate Paranormal Phenomena™

This best-selling book is ideal for beginners and advanced investigators who want to apply a more scientific approach. It contains a special scientific critical path graphic page to work from and a step-by-step guide to a complete paranormal investigation. It also tells you how to protect yourself from malevolent paranormal entities.

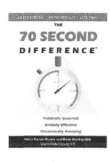

The 70 Second Difference™ - The Politically Incorrect, Occasionally Amusing, and Brutally Effective Guide to Strength, Fitness and Better Health
Approved by TWiEA – The World Isometric Exercise Association.
This is a science-based no-nonsense guide about the most efficient ways to exercise, build muscle and strength, and how lifestyle and dietary choices affect you. Just 70 seconds a day of focused science-based exercise can give you a total-body workout.

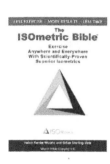

The ISOmetric Bible™ - Exercise Anywhere with Scientifically Proven Isometrics
Approved by TWiEA – The World Isometric Exercise Association.
A complete, practical, scientific, and user-friendly benchmark book about scientifically proven isometric exercise. No special equipment is needed for a total-body workout.

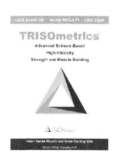

TRISOmetrics™ - Advanced Science-Based High-Intensity Strength and Muscle Building
Approved by TWiEA – The World Isometric Exercise Association.
An advanced, science-based high-intensity exercise system combining 3 scientifically proven techniques into a powerful new exercise system. It can be performed with or without equipment when travelling, or it can be used as part of a gym-based exercise routine.

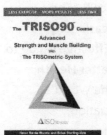

The TRISO90™ Course – Advanced Strength and Muscle Building with The TRISOmetrics™ System
Approved by TWiEA – The World Isometric Exercise Association.
A 90-day/12-week step-by-step highly advanced bodybuilding/shaping and strength-training exercise course. It combines three proven science-based principles It can be performed with or without equipment, or it can be used as part of a gym-based exercise routine.

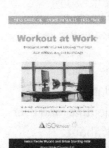

Workout at Work™ - Exercise at Work Without Anyone Even Knowing What You're Doing!
Approved by TWiEA – The World Isometric Exercise Association.
Time is the #1 reason why people do not exercise. The average person spends over 10 years of their life at a desk! With scientifically proven isometric exercise, you can exercise effectively at work without ever leaving your desk.

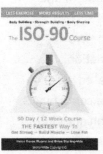

The ISO90™ Course – The 12-Week/90-Day Shape-up and Get Strong Course
Approved by TWiEA – The World Isometric Exercise Association.
A complete step-by-step 90-day/12-week isometric body shaping, bodybuilding, and strength-building course ideal for both beginners and advanced trainers.

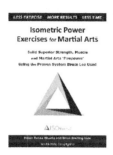

Isometric Power Exercises for Martial Arts™ - Build Superior Strength, Muscle and Martial Arts 'Firepower' Using the Proven System Bruce Lee Used
Approved by TWiEA – The World Isometric Exercise Association.
This book is a valuable resource for practical isometric exercises to build serious strength, muscle, and martial arts firepower.

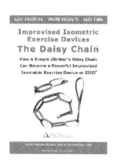

Improvised Isometric Exercise Devices - The Daisy Chain - How a Simple Climber's Daisy Chain Can Become a Powerful Improvised Isometric Exercise Device or IIED
Approved by TWiEA – The World Isometric Exercise Association.
Improvised Isometric Exercise Devices or IIEDs come in all shapes and sizes and are only limited by your imagination. This is a valuable resource listing practical exercises that can be performed as well as how to safely extend the daisy chain.

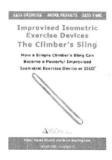

The Climber's Sling - How a Simple Climber's Sling Can Become a Powerful Improvised Isometric Device or IIED
Approved by TWiEA – The World Isometric Exercise Association.
IIEDs come in all shapes and sizes and are only limited by your imagination. This is a valuable resource listing practical isometric exercises that can be performed as well as how to safely extend the climber's sling.

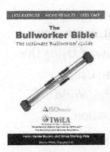

The Bullworker Bible™ The Ultimate Science-Based Guide to The Classic Personal Multi-Gym

Approved by TWiEA – The World Isometric Exercise Association. and the makers of The Bullworker. The original and best guide for all Bullworker® users and the companion book to The Bullworker 90™ Course. It is complete, science-based, and user-friendly showing how the device should be used to deliver maximum results. Also essential for the Steel Bow®.

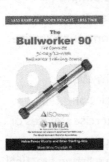

The Bullworker 90™ Course – The Ultimate Science-Based 12-Week/90-Day Get Strong and Grow Muscle Course Using the Classic Personal Multi-Gym

Approved by TWiEA – The World Isometric Exercise Association. and the makers of The Bullworker. A 90-day/12-week step-by-step course for all Bullworker® users and is the companion book to The Bullworker Bible™. Each week has a detailed note section, so you know exactly what to do and when to do it.

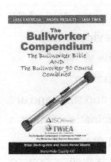

The Bullworker Compendium™ - The Bullworker Bible™ and The Bullworker90™ Course Combined

Approved by TWiEA – The World Isometric Exercise Association. and the makers of The Bullworker. The Bullworker Compendium™ combines both The Bullworker Bible™ and The Bullworker 90™ Course in a single huge book.

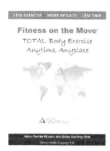

Fitness on the Move™ - Enjoy Gym-Quality Workout Sessions ANYWHERE!
Approved by TWiEA – The World Isometric Exercise Association.
This book lists practical exercises that can be performed while travelling almost anywhere and in any vehicle. If there is enough space to either sit down and/or stand upright, then you can perform a total-body workout!

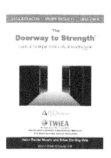

The Doorway to Strength™ - Turn a Door into a Strength-Building Multigym
Approved by TWiEA – The World Isometric Exercise Association.
It shows how a simple door, doorway, and frame can be used to create a multi-gym of exercises using the amazing Iso-Bow®. Required: 2 x Iso-Bows®, a solid door and frame, and a door wedge/stop.

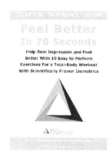

Feel Better In 70 Seconds™
Help Beat Depression and Feel Better With 10 Easy-to-Perform Exercises for a Total-Body Workout with Scientifically Proven Isometrics
Approved by TWiEA – The World Isometric Exercise Association.
Research shows that exercise can help to beat depression and can be done with little or no money, time, or space. 70 seconds of consecutive exercise is all that is needed to perform a 10-exercise total-body workout routine using the scientifically proven isometric exercise system. Required: 2 x Iso-Bows®,

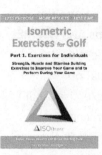

Isometric Exercises for Golf™ Part 1. Exercises for Individuals

Approved by TWiEA – The World Isometric Exercise Association.

Isometric exercises can be performed either during a game or practice and with just one exercise at each of the 18-holes then you get a total-body workout at the end of a game. The average golf club is a perfect Improvised Isometric Exercise Device or IIED. Part 1. is a resource guide of exercises for individuals and contains special exercises to increase the power of your swing.

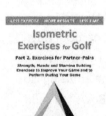

Isometric Exercises for Golf™ Part 2. Partner-Pairs

Approved by TWiEA – The World Isometric Exercise Association.

The companion to Book 1 is focused on exercises that are best performed in partnered pairs during a break, a game, or during practice sessions.

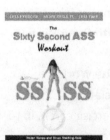

The Sixty Second ASS Workout™ - The Ultimate 60-Second Workout to Shape, Tone, Lift, and Give You the Backside You've Always Wanted

Approved by TWiEA – The World Isometric Exercise Association.

The fastest and most effective "ass" workout ever devised. Scientifically proven exercises deliver a no-nonsense time-efficient workout.

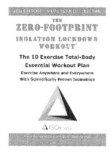
The Zero-Footprint Isolation Lockdown Workout - The 10 Exercise Total-Body Essential Workout Plan Exercise Anywhere and Everywhere with Scientifically Proven Isometrics
Approved by TWiEA – The World Isometric Exercise Association.

10 essential total-body exercises that can be performed anywhere, if you can stand and sit, then you can perform a powerful workout routine in as little as 70 seconds a day! NOTE: This is a variation of The 70 Second Difference™ workout.

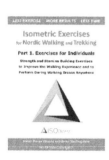
Isometric Exercises for Nordic Walking and Trekking™ - Part 1. Exercises for Individuals. Approved by TWiEA – The World Isometric Exercise Association. Perform gym-quality total-body isometric exercise routines during walk breaks almost anywhere using walking/trekking poles as an IIED or Improvised Isometric Exercise Device. Book 1. is a resource guide of exercises performed by individuals.

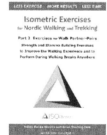
Isometric Exercises for Nordic Walking and Trekking™ - Part 2. Exercises for Walk Partner-Pairs
Approved by TWiEA – The World Isometric Exercise Association.

This is the companion to Book 1 and is focused on exercises that are best performed as a partner-pair, with a friend.

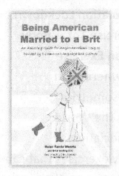
Being American Married to a Brit™ - An Amusing Guide for Anglo-American Couples Divided by a Common Language and Culture
A quirky, eye-opening, and fun-filled roller-coaster ride of how even the most basic everyday transatlantic conversations can bring laughter. It is dedicated to all transatlantic couples who are divided and confused by their common language.

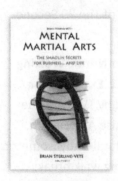
Mental Martial Arts™ - intellectual Life and Business Combat Skills
A system of intellectual languages and life-combat skills using the tactics and principles of physical martial arts. Learn how to verbally, and intellectually guide, channel, and redirect the energy of powerful people, and large organisations to achieve the outcomes that you desire.

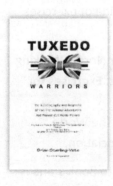
Tuxedo Warriors™
The companion book to both The Tuxedo Warrior book and the movie is the biography and autobiography of the iconic cult author, composer, and moviemaker Cliff Twemlow. It continues the story from where Cliff's book finishes and it is the most complete biography of Cliff Twemlow ever written from the late 70s to when he died. It is also the autobiography of Brian Sterling-Vete.

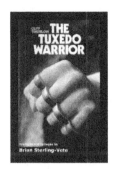
The Tuxedo Warrior™ by Cliff Twemlow – Prologue and epilogue by Brian Sterling-Vete. There are many ways in which a Doorman can gain respect. Numerous methods were applied to the principle. In my profession, every available technique must be utilised, depending on the situation and circumstances. Would-be transgressors either move off the premises and quietly acknowledge your diplomatic approach. Or, the other alternative whereby physical persuasion must be exercised, which either quells their pugilistic desires or it triggers their aggressive instincts, turning the whole incident into a bloody and violent encounter. 'The Tuxedo Warrior,' pulls no punches in its brawling, savage, colourful, and entertaining exposure of society's nightlife activities.

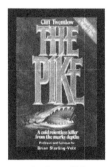
The Pike™ by Cliff Twemlow – Prologue and epilogue by Brian Sterling-Vete. ITS FIRST VICTIMS - A screeching swan... A fisherman overboard... A drunken woman...
One by one, the mysterious killer in Lake Windermere claims its terrified victims. Tearing off limbs with its monstrous teeth, horribly mutilating bodies. Fear sweeps the peaceful holiday resort when experts identify the creature as a giant pike…. A hellish creature with the strength to rupture boats, and the anger to attack them. But for some, the terror becomes a bonanza—the traders who cater to the gathering crowds of ghouls on the shore. And they will do anything to stop divers from finding the creature. Meanwhile, the ripples of bloodshed widen…. The Pike.

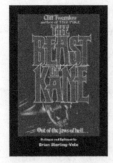

The Beast of Kane™ by Cliff Twemlow – Prologue and epilogue by Brian Sterling-Vete. When the Gordon Family open their door to a stray Elkhound, they unwittingly welcome in the forces of evil. For, according to the local priest, the huge dog is Satan himself, fulfilling an ancient prophecy. But no one will believe this warning... Even when sheep – and wolves – are mysteriously slaughtered. Even when frenzied pets turn on their owners. Even when Emily Forrest is savagely eaten alive – the first of many human victims. As winter tightens its icy grip on the remote town of Kane, its unprotected people must face an unearthly terror.

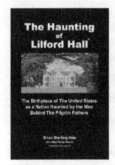

The Haunting of Lilford Hall™ - The Birthplace of the United States as a Nation Haunted by the Man Behind The Pilgrim Fathers. This is one of the most baffling cases ever recorded of paranormal activity experienced by multiple people between 2012 and 2013. Robert Browne is the man responsible for getting the Pilgrim Fathers to sail on The Mayflower in 1620 and it is believed that his ghost still haunts Lilford Hall.

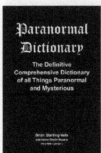

Paranormal Dictionary
A complete and comprehensive guide to all of the most common paranormal terminology, entities, and equipment used during investigations, plus, a few enduring mysteries for good measure. It is ideal for both new and experienced investigators.

Made in United States
North Haven, CT
22 February 2024